DBT

A Simple Guide to Cognitive Behavioral Therapy

(Practical Dbt Skills to Regain Total Control From
Fear Worries Anxiety)

Frank Adams

Published By Frank Adams

Frank Adams

DBT: A Simple Guide to Cognitive Behavioral Therapy (Practical Dbt Skills to Regain Total Control From Fear Worries Anxiety)

ISBN 978-1-77485-390-0

Legal & Disclaimer

The information contained in this book is not designed to replace or take the place of any form of medicine or professional medical advice. The information in this book has been provided for educational and entertainment purposes only.

The information contained in this book has been compiled from sources deemed reliable, and it is accurate to the best of the Author's knowledge; however, the Author cannot guarantee its accuracy and validity and cannot be held liable for any errors or omissions. Changes are periodically made to this book. You must consult your doctor or get professional medical advice before using any of the suggested remedies, techniques, or information in this book.

Upon using the information contained in this book, you agree to hold harmless the Author from and against any damages, costs, and expenses, including any legal fees potentially resulting from the application of any of the information provided by this guide. This

TABLE OF CONTENTS

Introduction

Anxiety disorders are common but they are also extremely manageable. The progress over the last 30 years of treatment for anxiety disorder is remarkable. Every one of these conditions responds to cognitive behavioral interventions that are specifically targeted to the specific issues. This is an amazing development for patients who suffer from these afflicting illnesses, for healthcare professionals who find ways to assist patients suffering from the same issues, as well as for the country's and world's health as a whole. This book is an important addition to the existing arsenal for medical professionals looking to offer their patients the best treatment.

Anger is a state of mind that captivates and is crucial. It can add passion and enthusiasm to our lives, providing us with a pulsing surge of energy that allows us to protect ourselves against oppression and injustice as well as defend our rights and confront those who abuse us. It can also be extremely annoying, due to its power as a sudden guest who disrupts the celebration. It could be a huge obstacle, and can put family relationships, our relationships and careers at risk. If we are passionate about or detest revenge, hold on to it or avoid it, rage is always enthralling. Therefore, you can be sure that it is something that we all have.

If you're studying this text, it's likely that you'll experiencing anger or anxiety, fear and depression. If that's the case, then you must know that you're not in isolation. The range of emotions can cause issues for a lot of people, which includes their jobs as well as relationships, and even physical health. A study revealed that 15% of participants scored very high on a test for aggression. A poll in 2003 found that more than a third of drivers of all ages said they were harassed or threatened when driving. Indeed, research on the effects of frustration has proven that extreme hostility and anger may increase one's risk of developing heart problems, cause relationships problems, create the barriers to working and hinder important objectives.

However, keep in mind that anger is one of your most powerful allies also. If someone hasn't been outraged by inequality or other people's unfair treatment and injustice, they are unlikely to decide to take action against injustices that affect society. At a personal level If someone is cruel to you regardless of whether you are feeling either anger or frustration the emotions that you feel will prompt you to take action to end the abuse. If you've been physically harmed by someone else, and you didn't feel angry in any way, you may not be able to defend yourself. Anger can be a powerful emotion that can be extremely empowering and motivating, giving you the energy you require to overcome obstacles, achieve, and push yourself to reach an objective. The objective, then isn't to get out of the anger but rather to be aware of it, and be able to manage it and utilize it to achieve what's crucial to you.

Over the last 20 years we've observed that when paired with scientifically validated treatments, the dialectical techniques that are derived from Buddhist philosophy show improvements of therapeutic outcomes. The initial evidence of this was in people suffering from personality disorders. However, today we can prove this is because these standard therapies improve the treatment of patients suffering from various disorders, but especially those who have an anxiety-related component.

How do one recover from anxiety, panic or phobias, PTSD and a tendency to worry to the point that one's ability to enjoy life is limited? The method involves finding out your current position on the road to recovery and recognizing that you desire more out of your life, and refusing to stop yourself from seeking help. Self-efficacy is what psychologists refer to as the determination to find a way around the obstacles that stand in your way.

The primary concept that is discussed in this book is mindfulness. A simple concept, its use in life is a recuperation structure. Like mediation it provides a means to be present as previous, ineffective coping strategies focus on the future. Mindfulness is a method of coping that promotes positive performance in the moment and creates an attitude of confidence that goes beyond what is normal. The practice is the key to developing mindfulness. Beginning with the most basic abilities, it is possible to advance easily to adapt mindfulness-based abilities to the most complicated and demanding situations and environments. The advantages of actively applying the techniques are significant changes in your perspective on what's important in their lives. If you are able to master these skills and you'll be able to accomplish things that you thought that you're not able to do.

What are the prospects for those with other cognitive abilities will be able to apply dialectical methods? The future is truly bright. Today, you utilize a notebook to guide your treatment and diagnoses, in the near future your treatment will be made available through the Internet. This World Wide Web presence would need care to be given immediately and precisely when you require it. For certain mental conditions, smartphones are already able to provide apps. There are many more that are in the process of growth. The current workbook is likely to be accessible through the ubiquitous smartphone with the release of its future version, so that tutorials, updates, and knowledge are readily accessible when you need they are, and at times when you'll require they. This is the ideal of the behavioral health system which includes therapy sessions in your home, workplace as well as social settings that are specifically designed for you. Support for social interactions will be offered in person or online when one is consistently successful in overcoming the obstacles that hinder enjoying life as well as achieving goals and developing a feeling of satisfaction.

Chapter 1: The History Of Dbt

DBT was developed in the early 1980s through The Dr. Marsha Linehan and colleagues. The term dialectics refers to being able to combine two opposing concepts. The primary objective for Dialectical therapy is foster a positive environment that promotes two opposite goals for individuals who "accept and change. It's an era in which two people differ on their views of an issue, however they attempt to find the truth using logic and reasoned arguments. The concept of a conceptual framework developed after the need for a solution emerged during the development of the most effective method of treating suicide sufferers.

Dialectics posits three things:

The inevitable change is here.

Everything is connected.

Two distinct thoughts can be combined for a better understanding in the direction of truth.

A validation program was provided by Linehan and emphasizes the importance of listening to patients with genuine care and concern. This non-verbal and verbal assistance will get maximum involvement from the patient. This aids in diagnosing and managing.

• Evaluate and explain the unspoken emotions of a person.

DBT Modules

Dialectical behavior therapy is comprised of four parts that include mindfulness the ability to tolerate distress, emotional regulation and interpersonal efficacy.

Module#1

Mindfulness

Mindfulness is the foundation on which all other skills is delivered through dialectical behavior treatment. It's a fundamental part of the concepts that underlie the science of the Dialectical Behavioral Treatment. It's the awareness, in the present moment that is free of judgment about your thoughts, feelings or physical sensations. The concept of mindfulness is derived and picked from the traditional religious practice but doesn't recite any metaphysical notion. Dialectical Behaviour Therapy trains people to be attentive, remaining in the present, not judging as well as observing one's behaviour and actions in a more holistic way. The process of mindfulness assists to assess what's going on outside by bringing people into the five sensory senses: smell, taste hearing, touch and smell. The process of mindfulness is highly driven and is based on acceptance. It's a technique that allows the person to accept the event, attaching to it, and has a bonded emotion to it. This means less stress prevails and this leads to less and less discomfort.

Acceptance and Change

The first phases of Dialectical Therapy are designed to introduce the patient to the concept of 'change and acceptance. The patient should be comfortable with the concept of therapy.

Prior to focusing on learning, one should be aware of the importance of radical learning. That means the student must confront both enjoyable and challenging situations without becoming too shrewd. Acceptance is linked to regularized emotions, and it is based on the foundation of a complete acceptance. When a person begins to recognize the idea of acceptance the idea of changing is never far away. The Dialectical Behavioral Therapy program includes five states of change which the therapist evaluates in accordance with the needs of the patient's. These are contemplation, pre-contemplation as well as preparation, action and the maintenance phase in descending order. In the initial stage of pre-contemplation, the patient doesn't know anything about their issue. In the second phase meditation, the patient is aware and is aware of the condition. In the third phase preparation, the person moves ahead to take preventive measures to see a therapist or find a solution through self. At the fourth stage, known as action that is self-explanatory the patient can take practical action and seeks treatment. In the final stage, called treatment, the patient reinforces the concept of change in order to reduce the chance of returning.

Module#2

Distress Tolerance

In the present our focus has shifted towards providing mental health services that may be the result of any negative event, i.e., broken families, relationship issues deaths, workplace problems, illnesses, terrorist attacks and a myriad of other kinds of tragic situations. This kind of problem is typically addressed through individuals-centered psychodynamic, psychoanalytic and narrative therapies and lessons from spiritual and metaphysical influencers.

The main focus of Dialectical Behavior Therapy is building and empowering oneself with the ability to bear and being able to face difficult situations effectively. The main goal of this therapy is to spot negative thoughts, feelings such as feelings, actions, and thoughts and then deal with them by learning the skills to transform it into positive thoughts patterns.

Six different types of treatment are available for DBT that deal with emotional distress. These skills include:

Skill 1

TIPP Skills

It's the fastest-growing and powerful skill of the ability to tolerate distress. It can reduce the symptoms instantly. Therapists nowadays advise patients who are emotional apprehensive and susceptible to self-harm to employ the TIPP technique. TIPP stands for Temperature breath-based breathing, intense exercise and paired relaxation of muscles.

When we're angered, our bodies feel hot. To combat this, wash your face with cool water, or relax in a space that is air conditioning. Altering your temperature can cause the body to lose heat and help cool your body on an physical as well as emotional levels.

* Twenty minutes of training at full intensity

* Engage in as intense exercise as you feel. An endurance of 50 meters, planks jumps, or another exercises until you've filled all of your motors. It has been proven scientifically that raising the oxygen level reduces stress levels.

* The pace of breathing. Sometimes, something as easy as controlling your breathing can help reduce the emotional stress. There are various breathing techniques that are used for calming your mind, including breathing it out or 'box breathing however, each one has four-second intervals. Breathe in for 4 seconds, holdfor four seconds, breath out and then hold for four seconds at each stage. A steady and calm breathing pattern reduces the need for fighting or reactions.

* Paired with muscle relaxation

* Science behind the concept of paired muscle relaxation is fascinating. If you contract your muscles, ease them and give it some time to relax and relax, your muscle will experience more relaxed than prior to, and you'll feel more at ease. Research has proven that a relaxed muscle has less need for oxygen, which means the heart rate and breath rate will drop.

Skill 2

Use ACCEPTS to distract you.

Skills used to free the person from a set of emotions that cause distress at present. The ACCEPT refers to the following: activities which contribute, make comparisons and push away thoughts, and feelings. These techniques are developed to allow a person to manage their emotions until the issue is resolved.

* Activities -- engaging in activities that people enjoy. One can keep themselves engaged in any kind of activity such as reading a book or calling a loved one and

making a banana shake and ironing your clothes. Any activity that keeps one engaged and free of negative thoughts can help.

* Contribute to --- helping and assisting others or the entire community by doing something to assist another person. The services offered can ease negative thoughts in a variety different ways. When offering services, one can take his mind off of the issues. We generally feel satisfied having helped someone as you aid a person struggling to overcome stress or depression. This can take the form of inviting your loved ones for dinner, washing the clothes of an acquaintance, cleaning up the home to assist your mother, wife or daughter or cooking for neighbours; all of these acts of kindness can aid a person in getting rid of negative thoughts.

* Comparisons -- the comparison of oneself to others in a bad state. It could be a look to the past where he struggled with emotional turmoil and apprehensions or

contemplating how one has the privilege of having an apartment and food, even though millions of people around the world are fighting to get a bite of bread and have no space to rest. The concept behind this isn't to make it easier to feel the burden of feeling, but to create an entirely new path to the issues one is experiencing in the present.

* Feelings- attempt to be different by stimulating the sense of humor. You can create completely different emotions from the present overwhelming feeling. If you're depressed Try taking an excursion in the park. If you're anxious look at images of puppy pictures. In short, giving an injection of different emotions aids in lessening the intensity of the emotions that overwhelm you.

* Push Awayby putting yourself in a second situation and temporarily let something else be your primary focus in your head. It's acceptable to put things aside when you are unable to manage it at the speed of. It is possible to shift your

attention on other things or thoughts, and return when you are ready to tackle the issue.

* Thoughts -- that keep your mind thinking about other things. It's about substituting negative thoughts with things which simultaneously stimulate your mind. It could be in the form of saying the alphabet or counting backwards or solving a problem. This shift of focus will help avoid personality-destructive behavior until you're in a position of getting emotional regulation.

"Sensation" do something that is filled by intensity. Utilizing five senses to soothe yourself in times of anxiety could be beneficial. Self-soothing can take place such as having a hot shower or listening to soothing music, eating your favourite food, or even watching a fascinating film. In simple terms any activity that is appealing to your senses could greatly help you overcome the negative circumstance.

Skill 3

Improve the moment

Skills are used to calm individuals in times of stress. The principal goal is to utilize positive mental images to get over or change the present troubling living situation. The abbreviation for this skill is IMPROVE.:

* I - stands for images, for example, contemplating a wonderful scene of an enjoyable relationship with a beloved and thinking that the negative emotions are disappearing. Imagine yourself facing a variety of complicated situations could provide you with the ability and the confidence to alter the outcome of your problem.

* M - can be used for creating or constructing the meaning from a difficult scenario.

* P stands for prayer. It could be directed towards God or any other higher force that seeks the power of God and being open to the present. Let go of your

struggles and request to be able to endure those moments a little longer.

* R stands to relax, and is achieved by deep breathing. This assists in calming the body's muscles that are large. It could take the form of listening to your favourite song, doing yoga or hot bath, a unwinding in a stroll while watching a film, or sipping a pina-colada. The goal is to immerse yourself in activities that help you to overcome the mental issues that you are facing.

* O is used to refer to something specific in a moment, meaning that one is able to remain neutral and focused on the present moment's activities. The goal is to remain present by letting the past and the future be remain in the same space.

* V is an abbreviation for vacation, meaning having a break from a challenging situation by imagining or doing something enjoyable. It can take the kind of thing as going to a beautiful location, turning off the television, not answering calls or just sitting in silence. After completing such an

activity the person comes back to the normal routine and is eager to face the challenges.

* E is for encouragement. It is achieved by interfacing with someone with a friendly and positive mannerthat can help them overcome stress and negative situations. It is not intended to be derived from outside sources. It can come from motivating yourself with a meaningful phrase to yourself, such as "all is all well."

Module#3

Emotional Regulation

Adults must control to regulate, manage, and control their emotions in a manner that is acceptable to others and also personally beneficial. The most common signs of emotional instability are when a person hasn't had the ability to control his emotions. When this happens they tend to perform or say things they regret or wish to control the emotions. Meditation or mindfulness and managing stress are just some of the techniques that can help to treat an individual and address negative thoughts patterns.

Apart from that however, these methods also tend to provide additional benefits like compassion, a sense of self-worth as well as a positive mood change. There are a variety of ways to impact a person's psychological situation, but this one tends to decrease the effect of them.

The regulation of emotions is comprised of three elements caused by emotions:

* Beginning actions.

* Facilitating actions

* Modelling response.

Emotional Regulatory Disorder

It's a condition of disorganized and ineffective ability to regulate and manage emotions visually. It's used to describe the deviated and poorly controlled spiritual reactions. The symptoms are as follows:

* Unpredicted and unintentional anger outbursts can be transmitted to someone who did not cause harm.

* Extreme discomfort and illness is not related to any type of medical issue and remains undiagnosed by doctors.

* Self-destructive behavior is characterized by the thoughts of suicide that are intense.

I'm struggling to find good social engagements

Attention dysregulation. The mind is stuck in the negative thought pattern.

* Insufficiency in self-control and hypersensitivity

The most challenging aspect of an illness is that it is accompanied by mental health problems like stress, anxiety or extreme mood polarities. The most popular treatment for EDD is called Dialectical Behavioral Therapy, which includes emotional assistance and cognitive techniques.

Reducing Emotional Vulnerability

The abbreviation for the initial technique to lessen the vulnerability of your emotions is "please learn to master."

The purpose of PL is to take charge of physical well-being and curing diseases.

E means having a balanced diet and abstaining from foods with high carbs.

A is for abstaining from alcohol and other substances that cause emotional instability.

S is to ensure that you get sufficient rest.

E is for regular exercises.

MASTER - points for everyday tasks that build competence and confidence.

The ability is developed to decrease the vulnerability of emotions by creating positive experiences to bring balance to life's negative aspects. People are encouraged take the positive aspects of their daily lives which they can reflect upon and appreciate.

Module#4

Effective Interpersonal Communication

The way we communicate can have a profound impact on the quality of our relationships. People who suffer from Dialectical Behaviour Therapy are taught the skills needed to start and build conversations with a thoughtful and mature approach instead of responding spontaneously to distress or stress. The main concepts in this program are the ability to request things and to deny them, when needed. This module is based on Dialectical Behaviour Therapy developer Dr. Marsha Linehan recognized three kinds of effects that need to be taken into account when discussing interpersonal interactions:

* Objective

* Relationship

* Self-respect

The three elements mentioned above must be considered in all situations. One is happier when an effective relationship is built around their top priority.

1. Objective effectiveness focuses on the end goal that the communication is aiming for, which generally results in tangible outcomes. Imagine a man is waiting for to hear from his wife during the time she is working late.

2. The term "relationship effectiveness" refers to the goal of having a non-conflict relationship. In this scenario the husband could place the emotional contagiousness of his wife and polyphony as his top priorities.

3. Self-esteem effectiveness could be the top priority If the patient feels that her absence from calling is insensitive to him. DBT employs acronyms to aid patients in remembering their capabilities.

DEAR MAN

is an acronym for an objectively effective The skills are listed below:

D - Describe: fully detail the situation.

E Express: Express your feelings, tell others what the situation makes you feel.

"A - "Assert": make wishes, say, what you'd like to have and what you would not like.

R - Reinforce: reaffirm the reason why this outcome is desired.

M is Mindful. remain present and present while focusing on the objective.

A - Look confident, with a confident face contact and tone and posture.

Negotiate: Be willing to negotiate and offer to receive while ensuring that each party has valid requirements.

GIVE is an acronym that refers to relationship efficiency:

G G Gentle Approach with a smooth, nice and gentle manner, avoid making rude remarks.

If I am interested, appear curious while listening to other person without causing interruption.

Verify: confirm and accept the other person's thoughts and feelings.

E is easy: act in an easy posture by softly smiling while using an elegant tone.

Then lastly, the Dialectical term used in behavioral therapy to describe self-respect efficacy is FAST.

F . Fairness: try to be fair to all people, including yourself, in order to avoid resentment.

A - Apologize: apologize for the minimumamount; make a statement only when it is appropriate.

The S-Stick: adhere to your core values and never compromise your dignity to achieve the goal you desire.

True: Be truthful and don't be apathetic to affect others.

The interpersonal skills taught by DBT improve the chances of a pleasant outcome, regardless of what the person's preference is for the ability to be relationships, objectivity and self-esteem for an interaction. When used correctly and effectively, the DEARMAN-GIVE-FAST skill can allow a person to express his needs in a clear manner without having to read their thoughts.

Components of DBT

Dialectical behavior therapy is an technique that therapists employ to concentrate on a patient's mental illness's emotional and social components to help treat it. It first came into use in cases where people suffering from Borderline Personality Disorder (BPD) attempted suicide. The method was employed to effectively treat these patients. Furthermore, DBT can also treat other disorders like addiction, depression, PTSD (Post Traumatic Stress disorder).

There are four fundamental elements of DBT:

1. Skills Training Group

2. Individual Treatment

3. DBT Telephone Coaching

4. Consultation Team

Skill Training Group

This method aims to improve the client's behavior skills by using various methods. It's similar to group therapy, however instead of discussing what they feel, they are taught how to manage their emotions successfully. The therapist will teach them strategies that help them improve their behavior abilities. Alongside giving them instruction that, the therapist also teaches them to use these strategies at home in their everyday life. This assists them in incorporating the most effective methods to help manage their disorder. The group therapy session lasts for about 2 hours each week. It is a 24 week therapy that is able to be repeated and extended to a full year program.

Every group has a schedule and is managed in a manner that is appropriate. The schedules are created to teach skills to the individual in a way that is effective. The skills are arranged according to the traits or skills the person is likely to miss in their character. Group sessions have proved to be a valuable part of Dialectical Therapy for Behavioral Issues.

Individual Treatment

Sometimes, the therapist may come across a person suffering from social phobia, or another similar disorder. These individuals are not able to be successfully treated in a group; therefore it is recommended to pursue individual therapy for these patients. Individual therapy helps the patient gain confidence and improve other abilities. This is a successful method as well as one that is sought-after by those who prefer privacy.

Chapter 2: Dialectical Behavior Therapy Overview

Dialectical Behavior Therapy (DBT) is one type of therapy that focuses on cognitive behavior. Its main goals are to teach people how to be present in the moment as well as adapt quickly to the pressures of life, manage emotions, and enhance relationships with other people.

The idea was first proposed to help people with Borderline personality disorders (BPD) however it is now being adapted to various conditions in which the patient has self-destructive behaviors, or struggles over emotional regulation such as for instance, alcohol abuse or eating disorders. It can also be employed to treat post-traumatic anxiety disorder (PTSD).

History

DBT was created in the latter part of 1980 through the late 1980s by Dr. Marsha Linehan and associates when they discovered the cognitive behavioral therapy (CBT) by itself didn't work exactly as it should in patients suffering from BPD. The Dr. Linehan and her group developed methods and created an intervention that met the needs of the new patients.

DBT is a philosophical method known as dialectics. Dialectics is based upon the notion that everything is composed of contrasting extremes. The changes occur when there is the presence of a "dialogue" between opposing forces or in more academic terms, the antithesis as well as synthesis, thesis, and antithesis.

The more specifically, dialectics asserts three fundamental assumptions:

Everything is interconnected.

* Change is gradual and inevitable.

* Opposites are able to be coordinated to provide a better understanding of the real world.

In DBT therapy, both the therapist as well as the patient attempt to discover the apparent inconsistency between self-acknowledgement and the need to bring about positive changes for the patient.

Another option offered to Linehan and her team was to gain approval. Linehan and her team discovered that with approval, along with the pressure for change, patients were likely to be involved and less likely to experience in a state of distress over changing. Therapists agree that the person's behavior "bode well" in the context of their interactions, but without agreeing that they're the most effective solution to the issue.

How It Works

DBT has evolved into an evidence-based approach to psychotherapy for a range of issues. When the patient is receiving DBT they are able to take part in three therapeutic environments;

* A setting where the individual is taught about their behavior capabilities through assignments for homework and role-playing the best ways for interaction with other people.

• Individual counseling with a certified expert in which the acquired behavioral capabilities are tailored to the individual's unique issues in life.

* Telephone training where the participant can reach their therapist between sessions for advice on dealing with the stress of a situation.

In DBT the therapists attend an interview group in order to help in managing their emotional demands of their patients. They can also help in navigating complicated and difficult situations.

Each therapeutic setting is governed by its guidelines and goals The underlying characteristics of DBT can be found in group capabilities psychotherapy for individuals, training as well as telephone coaching.

• Support and encouragement: you'll be guided to recognize your strengths and traits, and to create and utilize them.

* Behavior: You'll learn how to analyze any issue or harmful behavior patterns and

replace them with efficient and healthy behaviors.

* Cognitive: The focus will concentrate on changing your thoughts, beliefs and behaviors which aren't beneficial or productive.

Skills You'll acquire new abilities to enhance your abilities.

* Acceptance and transformation Learn how to accept and live with your emotions, life, and your own personal skills to assist you in making positive changes in your behaviour and interactions with others.

*Collaboration: You'll learn how to effectively communicate and work in group (therapist psychiatrist and Group therapist).

DBT Strategies

Participants in DBT learn how to alter their behavior by using four methods.

Core Mindfulness

Mindfulness-based abilities, which are perhaps the most important process in DBT is to teach you to focus on the present moment or "live now." In this way you will be able to figure out the best way to pay attention to the things that are happening inside your own mind (feelings thoughts, thoughts, emotions or sensations) and also things outside of your mind (what you experience, feel or feel, touch, and smell) in a non-judgmental manner. These skills will help in slowing down so that you can concentrate on healthier ways to cope with emotional turmoil. Mindfulness can help you in being quiet and refrain from engaging in negative thought patterns and uncontrollable behaviour

Example Exercise: Watch the Mindfulness Skills

Pay attention to your breathing. Notice the sensation to breathe in, and out. Watch your belly change in shape while you breathe.

Distress Tolerance

Distress tolerance teaches you to be aware of the situation in which you are currently. In addition you learn the best way to handle situations using four strategies that include self-soothing, enhancing the present moment, avoiding distractions and thinking about the advantages and drawbacks to not accepting anxiety. Through learning about distress tolerance strategies and techniques, you'll be able to anticipate beforehand for any unusual feelings and adjust to them from a more optimistic long-term perspective.

Go up and down the steps. If you're inside, walk outside. If you're seated, stand up and move around. The idea is to distract yourself by allowing your feelings to be a part of your body.

Effectiveness of Interpersonal Relationships

Interpersonal Effectiveness allows you to to be more assertive in relationships (for instance, communicating requirements as well as telling "no") while still keeping the relationship healthy and positive. This is accomplished by understanding how to listen and communicate effectively as well as manage difficult people and consider yourself as the other individuals.

Sample Exercise: GIVE

Make use of GIVE, abbreviation GIVE to enhance positive relationships and communication:

* Gentle: Do not be threatening or accuse anyone of judging or attacking

* Be interested: Show enthusiasm by listening well (don't interrupt your conversation)

* Validate: Accept the person's thoughts and feelings

* Simple Try to maintain an attitude of simplicity (smile and be lighthearted)

Emotion Regulation

The ability to regulate emotions gives you a variety of capabilities that allow one to better comprehend the sensational emotions. It helps you recognize from, identify, and alter your feelings. By recognizing and adjusting to intense negative emotions (for example, anger) you will be able to reduce your vulnerability to emotional outbursts and have more positive emotional experiences.

Sample Exercise: Opposite Action

Find out what you're feeling and then reverse the process. If you're feeling sad and wish to be away from family members take the opposite approach. Plan to visit loved ones , and continue to be active.

Is DBT the right choice for you?

Although the majority of research has focused on the efficacy of DBT for people suffering from borderline personality disorder , who struggle with thoughts of suicide or self-harm. DBT has also been used to treat a variety of mental health ailments, such as:

• Binge-eating disorder

* Attention-deficit/hyperactivity disorder (ADHD

* Bipolar disorder

* Generalized anxiety disorder

* Bulimia

* Major depression (including chronic depression resistant to treatment as well as major depression)

* Substance use disorder

* Post-traumatic Stress Disorder

If you're having self-destructive thoughts or thoughts, contact for help the National Suicide Prevention Lifeline at 1-800-273-8255 to get help from a qualified instructor. In the event that you, or your loved one or family member is in imminent danger, dial 911.

Researchers have also discovered that DBT is a viable option, paying no attention to gender, age or sexual orientation, as well as race or ethnicity. The best method to figure out whether DBT is right appropriate for you would be to talk with a professional in psychological wellbeing who will evaluate your medical conditions, your treatments history, and goals to determine the best method for you.

An Opinion From Verywell

If you believe that you or a family member might benefit from DBT or other forms of therapy, it's optimal to seek advice by a specialist or human services professional who is who are trained in this approach to treatment. DBT Therapists aren't always accessible.

Begin your search by using the Clinical Resource Directory maintained by the Behavioral Tech Association, an organization created by Dr. Linehan, to train emotional wellness specialists in DBT. The index lets you search by state for practitioners and projects that have completed DBT training through Behavioral Tech, LLC or the The Behavioral Clinical Research and Therapy clinics of the University of Washington. Another option is to ask your therapist, doctor, or another psychological health professional for a referral to someone who is knowledgeable about DBT.

Chapter 3: Introduction The Cognitive-Behavioral Approach

As mentioned previously, Cognitive-Behavioral Therapy positively influences the course of treatment for patients suffering from bipolar disorder.

Cognitive-Behavioral Therapy (CBT) has evolved over time It is actually one of the most effective psychotherapy methods that over time have come into existence and evolved into other forms of therapies. In 1955, Albert Ellis, American psychologist and author of the essay New Approaches to psychotherapy methods, introduced the therapy that was initially is known as Rational Therapy (RT), later on, over time, Rational-Emotive Therapy (RET) and eventually Rational-Emotive Behavior Therapy (REBT) the most current and updated definition. Ellis's unique method has led colleagues to be more interested in the irrational belief system, i.e. belief systems that were dysfunctional and appeared to have an adverse prognostic influence in various conditions.

Another method of cognitive behavior includes Acceptance and Commitment Therapy (ACT). ACT does not constitute a specific technique however, it is a set of principles. One of the interventions/objectives of the therapy is called diffusion, also called de-vitalization. The word "diffusion" in English is a dual meaning: "defuse" and "separation". The common thread in any kind of emotional distress is actually the merging of the virtual reality that is created by the mind of one's self.

A key character in the development of CBT is Aaron Beck who already in 1964, despite starting with the ideas of Ellis (which Beck then over time would develop, alter and even add new concepts) prefers to be described as a cognitive psychotherapist rather than a rationalist or rationalist.

Beck claimed that patients suffering from depression were identified through a cognitive triangle that consisted of a negative perspective of self and of the present as well as the future, and that this adversely affected the way that thoughts are organized. This cognitive triad was held in place by a dysfunctional thinking pattern, which when activated, weakened the patient's ability to take control of thoughts, negative thoughts and automatic thoughts.

The psychology of the cognitive revolution during the 50s and 1960s resulted in the creation of significant writings on the concept of personal constructs as well as in the field of rational cognition therapy by Ellis. At this time, Aaron Beck, during his training, began to investigate the psychological mechanisms that were observed in depression. He believed that emotions and behavior were controlled by cognitive processes at an unconscious level. Beck used his theories and methods for therapy initially with depression and later with disorders of anxiety, with astonishing clinical results. Furthermore, the application of some techniques for coping with anxiety has led to the treatment was, along with being thought of as an evolutionary form of behaviourism became known as Cognitive-Behavioral Therapy (CBT). This has led to the growth of cognitive psychotherapy throughout the 1970s, and its rebirth into the late 1980s. The theory can be seamlessly integrated with neuroscience to gain a better understanding of a variety of mental processes, both pathological and other. This is a reference to the collection of skills that are not sufficient to resolve problems. They are developed in CBT sessions:

"S: "Specify general problem" "('specify the general issue').

C: 'Collect information'.

1 "Identify reasons or trends".

E: "Examine options".

"N: "Narrow options and experiment".

C: "Date appears" ("compare data").

E"extension, revise, and replace'.

CBT is a combination of two highly efficient forms of psychotherapy The behavioral psychotherapy assists in change the way in which circumstances that can cause problems as well as the normal emotions and behavior reactions people experience in these situations. It helps to learn of new ways to react. It also assists in relaxing the both body and mind, in order to feel better and think about and make more informed decisions. Cognitive psychotherapy helps recognize certain patterns of thought that are based on fixed patterns of thinking (belief) and the interpretation of reality that occur in tandem with persistent and intense negative emotions that are interpreted as signs and root of the problem, to eliminate their imbalance, enrich the thought process, and integrate them with other thoughts that are more objective, or in other ways more beneficial to the overall wellbeing of the individual. It has been demonstrated to be highly beneficial for people suffering from bipolar disorder and depression, eating disorders, anxiety disorders (anorexia or bulimia), eating disorders that are uncontrollable) and stress-related disorders , insomnia and other sleep disorders.

A summary of the benefits that cognitive-behavioral therapy (CBT) include:

Practical and tangible: the objective is to solve of specific psychological issues. A few typical goals include the reduction of symptoms of depression, preventing anxiety attacks, encouraging connections with others, decreasing social isolation and so on.

Concentrated on "here and right now". CBT is focused on engaging all the resources of the patient and offering strategies that could be beneficial in removing him from the issue that can entrap the patient for a prolonged period regardless of the cause.

Short-term. CBT is a short-term therapy, as often as feasible. However the therapist is usually willing to declare the method ineffective if even partially positive results, analyzed by the patient themselves is not seen within a set quantity of therapy sessions. The time frame of therapy typically ranges from three to twelve months, typically each week.

Aims at Purpose. CBT is more purpose-driven than other types of treatment. The cognitive-behavioral therapy therapist, in actual fact, works with the patient to determine the goals of therapy, forming the diagnosis and establishing with the patient on the treatment plan which is tailored to the patient's needs during the initial sessions. The therapist also ensures regularly monitoring progress to ensure that the goals are being successfully achieved.

On. Both the patient as well as the therapist take part within the therapeutic process. The therapist attempts to instruct the patient information about his issues and the possible solutions. The patient, on the other hand is able to work outside of the therapy session to apply the methods learned in therapy by completing assignments given to him. In CBT the therapist plays an active role in solving the patient's problems, often intervening and sometimes becoming "psycho-educational".

Collaborative. The therapist and the patient collaborate to develop strategies that help the patient in solving their issues. CBT is actually a brief psychotherapy that is based on the collaboration of both the patient and the therapist. Both are engaged in identifying the particular methods of thinking that create the different issues.

Particularly specifically for Bipolar disorder, CBT is designed to assess the signs, the history of the condition and prior treatmentsas well as the coping strategies employed through a thorough evaluation. It's a plan to give accurate information regarding the symptoms that are associated with this disorder. It also provides information on their treatment and stages of treatment. Cognitive therapy is focused around the evaluation, monitoring and alteration of thinking styles that are dysfunctional and directing the patient to seek out concrete evidence and alternatives to hypotheses by analyzing the logic of deformed thoughts in relation to emotions, as well as thoughts that are related to depression and thoughts of anger, or excessively positive thoughts about depression; and the establishment of a consistent routine that assists the patient to develop strategies for self-monitoring and self-adjustment for emotional to plan their day to reduce the amount of things that could alter or decrease the intensity of their mood. The identification and modification of cognitions with strategies for cognitive restructuring that alter the dysfunctional automatic thoughts that are resistant to change, recognize their limitations, and develop an optimistic view into the near future. In this stage, the sessions are designed to modify the patterns of behavior that are non-adaptive by completing tasks that encourage the adaptive behaviour.

The guidelines developed in the American Psychiatric Association (APA) as per

Evidence Based Medicine, show that CBT is now the primary treatment option for a variety of mental disorders especially those with schizophrenia and bipolar disorder. CBT is the method which has the most experience for treating disorders of affect. Patient education is crucial to the effectiveness of the treatment. CBT can be utilized as a combination or monotherapy treatment for treatments for acute or preventative phases. The most important components of CBT-based psychotherapeutic treatments for Bipolar Disorder are:

information and understanding of the pathology that is personal to you and a more accurate assessment of personal risk that it poses.

self-monitoring regulator: modification of unadaptive behavior. Increased adherence to medications and treatments.

La mindfulness-based Cognitive Therapy

We are currently in the era of the third wave, or the third wave of cognitivism. It was first introduced in the 1990s and continues to develop (the beginning of the evidence-based therapies created in during the 50s, 1960s, and are today referred to "radical therapy for behavioral disorders" and the second was in the 1960s with the advent of cognitivism developed by Aaron Beck in the USA and ran up to the mid-90s).

To complete my research I've determined to develop a method which best fits my research questions and the results that form the result of this third wave. This strategy was designed specifically to treat depression symptoms and prevent return. It integrates current techniques for treating behavioral and cognitive issues and methods, while incorporating innovative aspects. The primary novelty that is the result of this third phase is embodied in Mindfulness the therapy that was created by its founder Jon Kabat Zinn in 1979 who came up with, realized and organized the possibility of using this technique in the treatment of chronic illnesses through an approach called

Mindfulnessand base Stress Reduction (MBSR), an alternative medicine program that was that was first developed by the University of Massachusetts. MBSR is also the cause of an increase in interest and the acceptance of mindfulness techniques to treat various conditions for both healthy and sick patients. Self-awareness techniques mindfulness, meditation, and meditation are "secular" methods that have received a lot of attention and recognition from the global scientific community. The methods that are derived from the traditional techniques of contemplation are being utilized in the contemporary practice without religious roots and spiritual significance. Meditation is the method that allows a person to reach self-awareness. Mindfulness is a type that is a form of Buddhist meditation. The word"meditation" comes in the Latin "meditari" meaning the practice of focusing on contemplation or contemplation. It's an awareness state that is constant of the present moment and not in the mental. A state of selfawarenessthat is quiet and completely healthy.

It is often referred to as a way of being aware of breath. The body in the Western culture. It was derived through Indian and Eastern practices, an enlightened mindset that is accomplished by turning your attention to the present moment, now and now. The primary goal is to pay attention at times to the body of one's, or to one's personal pleasant or unpleasant basic sensory experiences, like the sound of a hue or a bright spot to emotions such as sadness, anger, compassion towards things in the mind or to everyday actions like, for instance when washing dishes or doing an activity like pouring tea. The most important thing is to remain with a calm state that is not reactive but a state of being passive, allowing whatever happens. Psychologists who are cognitivists also employ this technique to change the root of negative thoughts in organic illnesses like cancer or psychiatric disorders such disorders such as depression. The most effective method to begin establishing this kind of awareness is to pay attention to the breath and concentrate on the breath. If thoughts do make their way to the brain, it's important to avoid judging them, and not be a follower, but to gradually bring focus back to the breath in constantity. The term "mindfulness" refers to the practice of Mindfulness in the field of psychology is often interpreted as consciousness of their behaviors, emotions, and mental states, and paying focus on the present every moment with an unprejudiced look and a predisposition to accept. Many studies over the past few years have examined how meditation can aid people to feel better after having been effectively treated for depression. when a patient is recovered from a depression episode, a little bit of depression can return regardless of the reason, which can trigger another round of traditional negative thoughts about depression that trigger physical sensations of fatigue, weakness or unfathomable suffering. The method could be in a position to stop the new episodes of depression. The simplicity of the way Mindfulness is integrated and Cognitive Psychotherapy has resulted in the development of a variety of methods of treatment that make usage of Mindfulness (MBCT, Mindfulness-Based Cognitive Therapy created by Teasdale, Segal and Williams; ACT, Acceptance and Commitment Therapy; DBT, Dialectical Behavior Therapy developed by Marsha Linehan).

It is believed that Mindfulness-Based Cognitive Therapy was developed in the late 90s. With it, we reclaim the importance of the body as well as the elimination of the Cartesian dualism between body and mind.

The theory behind MBCT is founded on the theory of differential activation that was developed by Teasdale in 1988. It suggests that people who have had a number of depression-related episodes are more susceptible to relapses and repeat episodes of depressive disorders, since even a mild dysphoric condition could trigger the same theories of depression that were largely untapped during the crisis. the likelihood of relapses is increased with each successive episode, as the new episodes of severe depression demand less and less of the trigger of stressors from outside.

It's a brand new approach for preventing the relapses that occur in bipolar and unipolar depression. They are specific programmes for patients that improve and develop awareness by using meditation techniques in conjunction with cognitive therapy methods. Through this, weaknesses which increase the risk of to relapses can be identified. The therapist will provide ways to tackle the issue and change dysfunctional thoughts to your benefit. The MBCT assists participants in understanding how their mind functions and to spot the signs that their mood is beginning to decline. It is designed to boost metacognitive capabilities by inducing people to change their ways of acting and living. This can help eliminate the connection between negative thoughts and negative moods that is normally activated. The participants are able to let go and experience with negative thoughts, moods and feelingswithout needing to fight them. The cultivation of awareness of the present and non-judgment allows people to break the circle of rumination and improve their kindness towards themselves and others, breaking the connection between the work that the brain does (ruminating about the past) and depression symptoms.

The practice may affect people on two levels. The first is via the immediate experience of their subjective state. This happens during meditation. It can include the subjective experience of calm as well as an easing or stopping of thoughts. This can result in greater clarity of perception. The second phase involves shifts in the way that thoughts are viewed emotions, thoughts and feelings. These changes bring about the feeling of greater calm and comfort, as well as increased perception of the world outside of the practice of meditation.

The MBCT provides eight weekly sessions lasting 2 hours each for an enclave that ranges from 8 to 15 participants.

The goal is to train patients to be more aware and to be more sensitive to their feelings, thoughts and bodily sensations. By practicing mindfulness exercises that include body scanning, yoga exercises, defocusing emotional by deep breathing techniques, closing-eye meditation, and stretching. These exercises aid the patient decentralize negative thoughts, reduce reactions to changes in the body's humor as well as to enhance the ability to fully be aware of the condition and remain in a state of the process of euthanasia.

In in addition to the therapy sessions suggested by therapists who specialize in the field, patients are encouraged to do exercises, like 40 minutes of meditation every day, and to practice the cognitive behavioral skills that are discussed in the sessions.

The primary difference between MBCT and traditional CBT has to do with the way

MBCT is designed to help patients learn how to be aware of the way they connect with their lives by focusing on awareness that is characterized by openness, curiosity , and acceptance, by developing a new perception of self-awareness and thinking as well as CBT will help patients change the dysfunctional thinking patterns of patients.

There is a National Institute for Clinical and Health Excellence (NICE) in Anglo-Saxon suggests this treatment for all patients who have suffered from at least two or more depression-related episodes. It has been demonstrated to be more efficient than maintenance doses of antidepressants to prevent an relapse in depression. It may also help decrease how severe symptoms are for those who are suffering from depression. It could also seem to decrease scores on the BDI (Beck Depression Inventory 3. In the case of Bipolar Disorder, research that have been conducted have demonstrated that the MBCT method results in an improvement in depression and anxiogenic symptoms, without an rise in manic symptoms. Mindfulness is an approach to health that has been proven effective. Mindfulness is also accepted by caregivers. In fact, it is an important idea to the the nursing profession. It can be applied to the wellbeing of nurses in the process of developing and long-term sustainability of the quality of the therapeutic care provided as well as for the advancement of overall health. It is essential for nurses that the health and self-care of the patient are in the education and research that he performs daily his primary objectives. It is crucial to figure out a way for everyone to be able to listen to the body language. Meditation can help you relax the mindand allows one to take in the moment of your day that are usually missed in the rush of chasing the sequence of things. It is the embodiment of all that nursing is about caring for others. It offers the chance to help the patient in every aspect of their work by personal learning about the profession, making the nurse more aware of the work he does as well as more sympathetic, which enhances his efficiency and concentration as well as educating the practice for the patient, helping to prevent diseases and promoting acceptance of a disease when there is one already.

Chapter 4: Standard Dialectical Therapy In Outpatient Settings

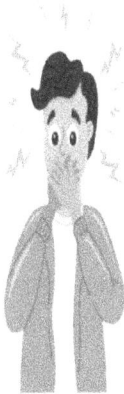

Therapy that is based in behavioral therapy (DBT) was initially developed as an experiment in outpatient settings, so what is the rationale to devote a whole section to outpatient DBT when writing an article that is a strong advocate for the usual DBT modifications? The most convincing explanation is that Linehan's manuals (1993a 1993a, 1993b) provide a wealth of information on DBT however the reader isn't given a lot of guidance on how to manage and maintain DBT as a part of a program. In addition, due to the highly influential books major advances were made in DBT in the context of outpatient care.

Additionally, there are further details on how to structure how to arrange the DBT treatment program in order to allow people to live a full and meaningful life (such as effectively resigning from the mental health field or working for a profit, and removing psychiatric impairment look up Comtois and co. (2006)).

The chapters have two major objectives: The first is to provide readers the knowledge and experience we've accumulated over the past decade when designing and advising about our DBT programs, and programs for a variety of other. We're here to help you "fast-track" the creation for your personal DBT program by providing all the details we've got.

I am a frequent speaker on the most commonly-held beliefs, as well as obstacles, difficulties and blunders when people implement DBT and give them tips on how to handle these problems.

Consider incorporating the criteria for inclusion and exclusion along with the possibility of insurance reimbursement in your DBT program by following our step-by step guidance. We also provide clear guidelines to create the DBT advanced program that focuses towards helping patients transition back to their lives as normal people and return to school and participate in more meaningful pursuits in everyday life.

Who Will Benefit from DBT?

Before you are able to begin offering the DBT program to customers You must make a crucial decision about the kind of clients you wish to serve. This will affect your hiring of staff, your location where you will house the program, the way you advertise and recruit clients, as well as how during the process of intake and evaluation you determine whether a client is a "match."

The requirements for admission can vary widely depending on the specifics of conditions like having the history of numerous suicide attempts and substantial emergency department and inpatient utilization, to less specific requirements like being a significant deficiency in their behavior due to the deregulation of emotion.

Certain organizations have rolled out DBT to all hard-to-treat, patients who use it frequently, due to the cost savings that DBT can bring to those suffering from BPD. Some professionals have considered the use of DBT during therapy sessions with people with BPD who "failed" using other methods.

To remain in the support of administrators as well as colleagues as well as the organisations that provide services for mental health clients with the highest value should be proven to be successful in clinical practice and savings in cost.

This could result from practicality. the factor that restricts client capabilities could be due to the fact that they have to pay for the treatment through their insurance or their insurance covers the treatment. When you are ready to proceed we suggest you adhere to two basic guidelines.

The first step is to use an evidence-based strategy to focus on the issue that the customer has to deal with. If the customer hasn't been treated for panic disorder It is not advisable to pursue DBT for the treatment of anxiety disorders, as DBT is less effective.

For bulimia or panic disorder or clients suffering from BPD, DBT should be the first line of treatment, as DBT is specifically designed to tackle various conditions. In this instance it is possible that DBT is chosen for a specific client who has certain behaviors that block the treatment from being successful regardless of whether the person suffers from BPD. This could be due to treatments that have failed previously or the availability of novel treatment options. Also, be careful.

Find the best place to begin DBT program development.

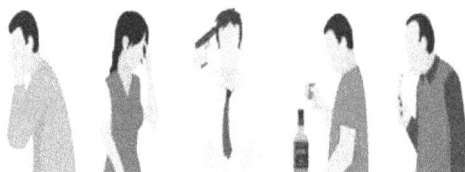

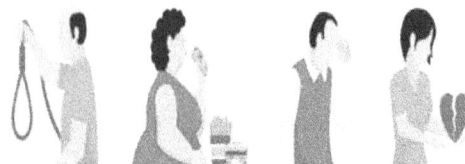

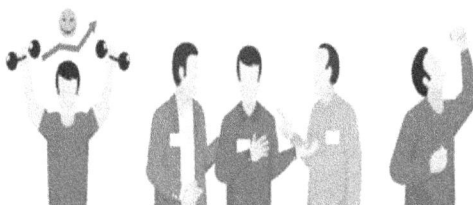

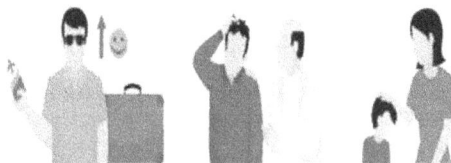

You'll have a range of choices concerning the place for your DBT program, regardless of whether you're an audiologist or working in a public-sector firm. What amount of DBT the clinician handles on cases can affect the methodology used to train healthcare professionals on DBT adhesion.

Certain organizations would like to have all the clinicians within their organization understand and be willing to employ DBT to those who have been recommended for treatment by a physician who has diagnosed BPD. The second option is for therapists who will take on treating the clients of the agency suffering from BPD and also serve as part of the DBT team.

Another way of thinking about it is that private practitioners dedicate themselves and their practices to helping patients suffering from BPD with DBT. Some patients with BPD is the only thing that independent practitioners can treat with DBT and, as such, they create a separate practice or join with other independent practitioners to design an DBT program.

In order to determine whether the DBT program will allow sharing of staff with other agencies it is essential to be aware of the way DBT programs are organized. It is also essential to know that having another job with more rewards, or having a less number of customers who are difficult to treat can reduce the exhaustion associated with work.

This means that the institution's DBT program may suffer in the event that it is dependent on expectations, which include events, further training and similar. Physicians are also faced with the added challenge of dealing with clients who have very different treatment strategies according to the organization or group.

If this is the case it's important to revise policies to give the DBT team with a distinct identity as well as the ability to work within the framework. The 60 to 120-minute weekly meeting with the team has an enormous impact on everything that takes place in the DBT office.

Another way to tackle this issue is to find out whether DBT clients are willing to work with DBT staff in any way regardless of whether they do it in part and in the majority or in a partial way. Akin as a partial model an incomplete model suggests that a certain portion of the care of the client is taken care of through members of the DBT team, while another team taking care of other aspects. similar to a primary model a primary model signifies that the main accountability for the client lies to that of the DBT group, and the other teams as aides.

A particular model will ensure that the treatment for the patient is carried out by DBT practitioners, even though they may be in contact with different types of health professionals. DBT teams are typically under-staffed and the significance for each DBT treatment option requires the requirement of only one therapist and team in order for DBT to work.

When crisis intervention is handled by anyone different from members of the DBT team, it's unlikely that a partial approach is in place. There could be a dispute in cases of suicide or having issues that are hard to resolve because there are multiple treatment teams and the members on each team have the same responsibility.

Primary models are ideal for patients as they provide patients with a range of services the DBT team is not able to provide for example, financial, residential, or professional help. Many people believe they are DBT is more complex than it actually is.

If asked if this method (as described within this document) could benefit frontline staff the therapists (seeking ways to deal with the most difficult situations) emphasize their involvement as the ones that initiated and support the growth of the program.

A lot of students who graduate from educational programs that are linked to

DBT decide to join the DBT team to be taught about the procedure. This is a way to encourage students to be DBT interns, and also encourages more students to be DBT students. As they search for opportunities in academic or clinical fields, students are aware of the value of this particular experience.

Incentivizing new graduates and other specialists who are part of an DBT team is extremely inspiring, especially since they've gained access to the panels through which insurance companies send patients (e.g. panels of therapists that have been approved by the insurance company to whom insurance companies make referrals). This gives them access to an existing referral database, in addition to a steady stream of income.

DBT programs typically have to be concerned about keeping skilled and highly educated DBT therapists, who could be scarce. Because of their training and expertise in the field of DBT is considered highly competitive in the job market, especially for job laterals or promotions that relate to the development or execution of an DBT event.

Although a small percentage of people would prefer to open up their private practice, others might prefer to begin an informal group practice instead. Retention of employees is the best chance to advance and be promoted Therefore, encouraging this expansion through the development of employees and plans for promotion is among the best ways to boost loyalty among employees.

Consultation with the Client

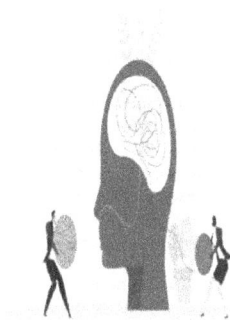

Also, observing your boundaries is a crucial part of controlling your emotions, and the DBT concept of consulting the client is a fantastic job in assisting lower levels of emotional exhaustion, as well as increased efficiency in therapy.

Although intervention could or might not be a part of the role of a Therapist, in essence, consultation implies that the job for therapists is educate the client to communicate with others, not acting on behalf of the patient, or instructing others on how to communicate with the client.

Customers must be included in this decision making process and not only you. Many people could fall into this category such as family members as well as other medical professionals and other medical professionals, and so on. An example will illustrate this concept: When Julie just began attending an DBT skills group in her local hospital Julie is 27 years old and is having trouble controlling her emotions. Her therapist suggested that DBT techniques could be beneficial to her.

But, Julie, who was continuing to go through her own treatment at that time informed her therapy therapist that she was considering about removing herself from the group due to feeling that the load was too heavy. Without an DBT Therapist, someone who isn't an DBT specialist may speak to the facilitator of the group about the issue. DBT Therapists begin by having a consult with the client prior to discussing the issue with the client, and then helping the client develop and apply techniques to cope to enable the client to speak on her own in subsequent sessions.

It could happen as this It is the job of every DBT Therapist to provide advice on how to deal with the client. A lot of times, clients place expectations on their therapists to advocate to have them admitted to a hospital when they're in suicidal.

The DBT Therapist will instead work with the client using the skills she has acquired to fulfill her requirements. There is also an expectation of an outside expert in the event when a doctor is calling to inform you that the patient would have to be discharged from the hospital and requesting what you should do with her.

According to Linehan (1993a) stated as the primary guideline for therapists is to employ conventional techniques. If I use the phrase "in another way," I want to highlight that clients' difficulties controlling their emotions isn't typically going to cause changes in the world around them. Instead it is the individual's duty to control their emotions.

If I'm working with teens that parents want to support them, I often come into this issue. I say that this isn't a part of my job as a parent may want to talk with me, but with the adolescent absent. If you have something at something to say you must take the client with you to ensure that your message is heard.

If a parent contacts me on the phone I inform the customer beforehand about the specifics about the call. Communication that is sensitive to emotions is essential when dealing with family members and friends of your clients. However, your clients need to learn to communicate effectively and handle situations like those on their own and you should help them through this process.

The purpose of providing consultation it is about teaching children skills in problem solving that they might not have learned to help them develop their independence. Instead of being dependent on others to do the work for them, consultation empowers people to be responsible for their own lives.

Things that interfere with therapy

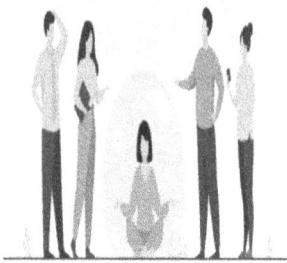

In order to discuss the behaviors which are the most detrimental in treatment. We'll begin by discussing the most damaging and move on to the most beneficial. There are a variety of different behaviors that can be employed and utilized by therapists and clients. If you're in the process of planning for your own session, you must be aware of this.

If a therapist or client delays or cancels appointments, they're not prepared for the sessions they are scheduled. It could be as simple as therapists putting too much pressure on their clients and shaming their clients or helping clients to maintain the unhealthy habits they have developed as well as the therapist or client ignoring key issues in therapy.

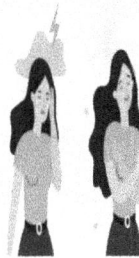

Certain behaviors that affect treatment can cause damage. For instance, a therapy therapist not being aware of the client's limitations or the client's threat to himself or herself.

Behaviours that affect the quality Of Life

In private sessions, the final item on the agenda will be to tackle habits that have a negative impact on their life quality. This could include anxiety, mood or addiction issues It could also cover things like inadequate financial or housing options as well as insufficient social support or possibly trauma or trauma-related issues.

This can be a challenge because people suffering from emotion dysregulation are often faced with several additional issues throughout their lives. Linscheer's advice (1993a) are as follows: tackle the immediate issues like getting a place to live or enrolling in rehabilitation first, then tackle more manageable issues and save the more challenging ones until the future; and lastly arrange your behavior to meet two other goals.

Chapter 5: The Wise Mind Accepts

The Wise Mind is among the three mental models that are taught in DBT. This is the best way to integrate your rational considerations and your emotions to be more natural and balanced approach to handle difficult situations.

Here is a useful DBT tool that allows you to develop the capability of diversion to ensure to operate in Wise Mind constantly often. When you're able to master it the technique, you can make this technique part of your daily routine. Its abbreviation Wise Mind Accepts causes you to remember how to utilize gradually enjoyable exercises to reduce negative and stressful thoughts.

Engage in activities to distract you

You can escape from the agitation of thoughts by engaging in exercise routines that catch your attention. Think about things you could do if not worried, and then try to take them on. Take a trip to the gym and finishing a crossword or watching a film, looking through your closet to find things you can donate to charity, taking an excursion, or taking part in a pastime that you enjoy. It doesn't matter the way you go about it so long as it's an effective activity, and it takes the mind away from negative aspects. Be aware that if you select an initiative that involves others, you should avoid talking about the issue. The idea is to do distractions to keep your mind away from the negative thoughts.

Do not distract yourself by giving

You can distract yourself by contributing towards the life of other people. Helping out others generally, it will be more relaxing and accommodating when you are doing some exercise for you. Contributions may include helping out with an organization or monitoring your friend, cooking a meal for an elderly person or helping your sister with painting her lounge or anything else that you do for someone else that takes you out of the disappointments.

You can distract yourself by comparing

Take a break by thinking about those who have been more regrettable in their lives than you. You can also see times that were more than you've ever experienced in your life. This will allow you to feel immense satisfaction with the present. The point isn't to deny the way you feel, but rather to help you place your circumstances in a different the perspective of others. The method of looking at the situation is to recognize situations that are more traumatic than yours.

Distract yourself with inverse emotions

Take part in exercises that create emotions that are the opposite of the emotions you're momentarily experiencing. If you're feeling angry, attempt to put an impromptu parody onto the DVD player , and you'll be able to spend the next few hours laughing. You can try singing or dancing in a mood of despair. On the other hand perhaps, you can watch someone doing sky diving or doing something risky when you're scared or anxious. The idea is to fill yourself with exercise that encourage you to experience the opposite feeling.

You can distract yourself by pushing away

This technique allows you to make negative thoughts go crazy by thinking about leaving the scene. It is important to allow yourself acknowledge that there is a problem, however, you should be able to take care of it nearer the time. It's not an attempt to avoid the major issues however it permits you to choose from the issue to receive some temporary help. One way to effectively use this technique is to imagine an imaginary wall between you and the scenario. Imagine that the wall is separating you from the case. It is also possible to try to imagine that you're pushing to the button that controls the volume on the case in order to ensure to smaller and smaller until you'll never be able to hear it. It is possible to imagine moving the problem into the cabinet of a different room where it will remain until you're in a better position to handle it. This method will give you a brief assistance so to get through any crisis or emotional apprehension.

Think about distractions

Consider entertaining your thoughts by imagining non-biased thoughts that aren't connected to your current circumstance. If you're stuffed with additional evidence, there's no room to continue the negative thoughts. You could consider giving the tiles a go on the floor, and imagine new furniture to your house, and speculating on the most popular shade of every child who passes through the gym, or calculating maths estimations in your head. This can help you avoid thinking about pain-inducing circumstances.
Use Sensations to distract you.

It is also possible to engage yourself by focusing on physical and significant sensations. Some of the exercises you can attempt include placing an ice cube over your neck and washing your hair and drinking a hot drink or listening the loudest music you can, putting an elastic band around your wrist, deciding on an air blower to blow into your eyes, or going swimming in cold water. Engaging in a variety of physical sensations will allow you to increase the energy in your body , and your mind and emotions will follow it. The strong impressions will help you get rid of the pain of your current circumstance. This is likely to be one of the best method to be "unstuck" during an emergency.

Wise Minds is a method that many people find helpful in everyday life. It lets you apply an ever-changing approach to confront difficult situations. This method teaches you how to utilize distraction when faced with situations that are beyond your control. What is most important regardless of the situation it is important to know that this tool will help you lower your emotional stress while combating harmful and unhelpful behaviors that could be damaging to your health. It is possible to get acquainted with Wise Mind ACCEPTS and other DBT methods by contacting someone who has knowledge of the discipline of Dialectical

Therapy. A quick internet search will provide you with an impressive list of practitioners in your area. There are as well DBT exercises manuals available to request on Amazon or available in your local bookshop.

How can you control your mind during DBT?

Mindfulness is at the heart the Dialectical Behavior therapy, which is a CBT treatment for pervasive emotional control issues. Each DBT group of skills begins by focusing on mindfulness. Each skill is dependent on the presence of mind. When trying to figure out what went wrong in your day, or when something goes right there is mindfulness involved. The reason why mindfulness is so important in DBT It is often not understood.

Treatment for emotional dysregulation is known as Dialectical Behavior Therapy. People are often affected by their emotions through seemingly insignificant or minor instances, not because of the actual events rather than the opinions people make about the game. You may, for instance, be employed in a job where you're generally happy in. It could be working in an apparel shop. You love clothes and you love connecting with others and so it seems to be a perfect combination. The one thing you do not want to do in any way is to fold clothes. You believe it's exhausting. You may have to fold your clothes for about 30 minutes in a 6-hour shift, but that's only an insignificant portion of your job. It is possible that when you refold your clothes and fold them, your brain begins to make all kinds of negative choices about the collapse of your clothes. "This is awful." "What is a waste in precious time." "This seems a stupid idea." "This task is awful." Instead of spending your energy in collapsing the clothing, your mind is consumed with thinking about to you all kinds of gruesome stories of this job, and could cause feelings like displeasure, anger, even despair.

The worst part is that these feelings have a way to influence the rest of the time. In contrast to having to endure thirty minutes of a painful task, you go through all day feeling awful taking a decision on everything you do in a negative way, and then feeling worse frequently. Being miserable throughout the time, more days than not, is extremely uncomfortable; you start making thoughts regarding your mood and conclude, "I can't take this for any longer." Then, what began as a minor incident has resulted in a great deal of misery.

Mind management

I was given 30 seconds to introduce myself and what I did. This is known as the lift pitch, and it's definitely not so easy as you think, particularly when your specialty is mind management. After observing how a handful of people were trying to finish their presentation in just 5 minutes, not forgetting the time limit of 30 seconds. It was suggested to use the quick-little recipe to help others by being the next one and stayed and said:

"I assist individuals in achieving their goals and make positive improvements in their lives and business through the management of their thoughts."

It worked because everyone went "oh" and were eager to understand what mean, what's mind management, and how do you do that.

And it made me think that it's been a long time since we've had a discussion about the things we actually do , or the reasoning behind what we do.

We're going to take advantage of that privilege by going back to the basics and pondering what is the most fundamental thing that supports everything We do here in Brilliant Living HQ. This is also the subject in my Changeability book, and it is the basis of the whole Changeability method and practice, as well as Brilliant Living tools.

Mind management: What exactly is it?

The key question is: What is mind-management and why does the world require it. It is at the most basic level the concept of mind management is connected to the management of your mind.

It's possible that it's not saying too much, or more often as it's an idiom, something that's identical twice - there's an appropriate term for it redundancy!

Mind management is entwined to managing your mind. We're affected by the entire thoughts.

The tagline we use in our office at Brilliant Living HQ is "Mind management to have the best time in your business and life maybe it was prior to the time we updated our website in recent times We thought that our logo was more appealing without it, however, perhaps we should reintroduce it to let people know what the message is!

The strapline for the podcast (and in the Changeability book) is "Manage Your mind - change your life.'

The reason why the focus is on the mind - what is at the root of it?

The management of your mind is the ability to manage your thoughts. that you are able to:

"Bridge the incredible power of your mind and allow you to achieve what you want from your life.'

So, you are able to refining or prepare your thoughts to have the right choice to turn your dislikes to what you like and achieve your goals and be free of limitations.

"The state of your existence is an impression of the perspective you have." -- Wayne W. Dyer.

It's a good starting point however, would we be in a position to further define it and look at the different elements of'mind management' to come up with an accurate definition?

What is the best way to describe the mind-management process?

The Business Dictionary defines management as:

"The co-ordination and coordination of activities of a company in order to reach specific goals."

The Merriam-Webster dictionary has a valuable additional dimension, which defines management as:

"The ability or act of controlling and making the business's choices."

If we put these definitions in conjunction and replace business with the same cognizance, we can think of:

"Mind management - The practice or demonstration of managing, sorting and planning exercises of the mind in order to (settle on the best options to) meet a specified goal."

This assumes that you've officially identified what you would like in your life and you have a vision of your clearly defined targets (objectives) and the steps you must take to achieve these.

For us this is the place where it usually starts by defining your goals - as there are clear mind-management benefits to doing this, and utilizing the energy of your brain and mind to allow you to achieve those goals and progress you desire. The first step is to establish your goal and motivation, which should be in line with the vision or goals you have set.

While under supervision. The next stage is currently in the works.

The Mind

There are two distinct parts of the mind: the intuitive and the conscious.

The conscious, which is the part we're conscious of, for instance when you're focusing on this, or when that you're having about what you'd like for dinner or drinks, or the things you're doing afterward or reacting to the sounds you're hearing. It's what we think of and are aware of. We , generally take it as "this is me," but there's much greater to your life than this.

Your conscious personality is the hints of something far more important because beneath it's what's commonly referred to as your mind, that part that is below the conscious part of you. We think of it as being beneath when thinking about an icy mass however it's not submerged (as in submerged and submerged) as long as we're is not observing it. Another name - that is more likely to be becoming more precise - is not.

This is what we're unaware of, however, it keeps us alive as it accomplishes a large range of activities without our conscious awareness of it.

When combined both of these parts of your brain create what's really an information-preparing system, that's goal is to keep you productive and active.

The brain, and the brain

When we speak of our minds, we're using the term to describe the various aspects that happen within our cerebrum. The majority of people use the two terms in reverse, however they're by no possibility quite alike.

There are various physical parts of your brain that are easily visible in any sketch of the brain. However, your brain is the one that is inside the organ of your body. The account you have is the place where consciousness and your personality are.

It's similar to the software that runs on a PC. Brain is the instrument and the brain is the device. However, it's not as clear as it appears because your thoughts are the result of your experience and your understandings and emotions. As a result, it's getting more and more blended.

Most brains have neuron cells (called neurons) which are connected via neurotransmitters. This is how thoughts shape.

These neural systems , or pathways can be strengthened through redundancy. In the same way, these pathways could be affected, either intentionally or unknowingly and strengthened by the things we do, and by the influence of our lives, and by memories, convictions and values we've stored in our minds.

It's not just one of the features or characteristics of the way that your mind works It's also a reason to desire to manage your mind.

Conscious and Unconscious Mind

If I am talking about blind procedures, they are the processes that you carry out and aren't aware of, which aren't even apparent to you. Anything that you're not aware of immediately is considered to be unconscious. Instinctive actions could be that are as easy as breathing or lifting your arms, and it can be as baffling as getting to work and not crash! Unaware techniques include ways of thinking, like recall of recollections facts, beliefs, and emotions.

Consciousness is the ability to act and reflections that you think about with intention. For instance, your comprehension of the terms you're reading at the moment, your estimations, organizing and executing actions.

Think about the mind-management capabilities required to become an exceptional leader, or the best tennis player. World-class tennis players are able to manage and control their emotions which is why they play the highest quality tennis when the pressure is most critical. They are able, by just watching the throw of the ball onto the server of an opponent or the position of their bodies, their backswing, to determine where the ball will be able to react and deliver an appearance within a matter of minutes. They aren't able to in any way, form or form do all this intentionally is it? A portion of it is conscious however most of it is in a state of obliviousness.

Leaders who are successful know what to do and what to say under extreme pressure to ensure a successful communication and result. They can be awe-inspiring at many moments at any given moment, yet they are able to be quiet and decisive. It's not just down to their activities or thoughts, but rather a mix of conscious and unconscious and almost instinctual reactions.

It has been stated on numerous times that the winner from the 100m Olympic gold medal wins the event before they start jumping on the first squares. I believe this to be true and is an amicable blend of cognitive considerations and tasks with non-conscious procedures that create the difference between joy, achievement and world-class execution.

Your future happiness and success

If you're not seeing the results you want in your life, or if you have actions that aren't helping your self-esteem, or you're not a jolly participant in your discussions and you want to be the top in the world in your area, then your response should be equivalent of enhancing your management of your mind. Focus on your inner world to create your external achievements. Make sure you have the perfect union between your subconscious brain and conscious.

How can you manage your views and be the master Of Your Brain?

Your brain is the most powerful resource you can have in creating the positive within your life. However, If it's not properly utilized can be the most harmful ability in your life.

Your mind, specifically, your perceptions affect your perception and, consequently, your understanding of the world as it is.

I've heard that the average person has 70,000 thoughts a day. That's quite a number, especially in the case of ineffective thoughts or self-harming and an unproductive waste of time.

It is possible to give your thoughts an opportunity to become wild but why do you think it is? It's your mind, your thoughts. Would you be a good chance to gain your power back? Would it be a mistake to think that it's not the best chance to control your life?

You can be the one who is consistently, purposefully thinking of your thoughts. Make yourself an expert in your thoughts.

When you shift your thinking then you'll be able to increase your emotions too and also get rid of the triggers that trigger the emotions. These results will provide you with a greater level of peace in your thoughts.

There are some thoughts that aren't just my own preference or the result of my reconstruction. I am the sole source of my thoughts, and as such, right now, my mind is peaceful. It is possible for you to be as well!

Chapter 6: Tip And Strategies To Improve Your Marriage Using Dbt

The Emotional Dysregulation System and the Emotional Understanding

The emotional system of our body is complex system that is composed of numerous components.

Take a look at the video below. Ella is feeling an uneasy feeling in her stomach and a stiffness in her mouth and clenching of her jaw muscles when she realizes that Josh isn't changing the toilet paper following an exhausting day at work. The flurry of stimuli that she experiences is what she describes as "rage."

The reflections she makes about Josh are also a part of the story. Her words are a narrative which goes like the following: "I can't bear how selfish Josh has become... whoa whoa, whoa Whoa I can't bear it, and he's just similar to his rude brother." Her emotions unfold as the intensity of her feelings increases as she gazes at the toilet paper roll that is empty. The stomach gets tighter, and the discomfort in her throat increases. "I am not sure the reason I got married to with him" the woman says in her head, "and he didn't seem to love me even though we were in an evening of love." It's not clear why I bother to speak to his... It's pointless.' More "anger."

Josh arrives in the living area, exuberant with excitement about his forthcoming vacation. He extends his arms to Ella and is eager to hug her and share travel details with her. He slams her away with her expression and he says, "What the hell is going on that you are doing... it's just that you have to be calm," and she retaliates with an insulting name and he responds with a more insulting name. The volume is increased by around ten decibels. Then their heart rate, blood pressure and adrenaline increase, culminating in Ella crying out of the room , crying and Josh screaming. It's a great relief! And, even more amazing is that all of this takes place in just a few seconds and, if not more.

How do you define mindfulness?

Mindfulness is the practice of being present in the moment instead of worrying about the past or looking ahead. Because we spend a lot of time worrying about the future or dwelling about the past, a lot of us don't seem to be living our lives to the fullest. We're distracted and disconnected from us, our environment and others due to our busy lives.

You don't need to do it in a yoga class or even when you meditate. Mindfulness is the act to look at all the things that we do, be it eating dinner or weeding the lawn. By slowing down and focusing on only one thing at a given time can help us develop the habit of mindfulness. It is more likely that we will notice the small details that could otherwise go unnoticed or assumed as normal because we employ all five senses. If we're attentive and aware, we can notice the little things in life like the bright light shining on our faces, or the crisp, clean sheets that we sleep on.

Be assured that mindfulness won't appear to be a natural thing for you. Mindfulness is described as practice or "practice" since it is a process that requires regular practice. We are accustomed to multitasking, working in multiple tasks, and scheduling our time. These are the two opposites of mindfulness. Mindfulness can help us have a more enjoyment in our lives. We are able to witness all kinds of events - and our own personal aspects by remaining present and grounded.

• Connect to yourself

Mindfulness can help us gain an understanding of oneself. We are prone to look for solutions that are outside of us when the most effective way to find out the person we really have become and the things we really need is to take a look within. It's not that there's no wisdom within ourselves, but the truth is that we're constantly cut away from ourselves. We're constantly intoxicated through alcohol, food drugs, technology and even pornography, we do not feel what we're going through or what we require. These are the simple solutions that we can turn to when down. They're easy ways to help us find comfort and distract our minds from our problems and emotions. We can discover solutions to our issues since we're mindful, so we are able to see the larger view; we are able to allow our minds to be open to new ideas rather than becoming entangled in old thought routines.

Mindfulness as a tool to Accept Self-Care

Because we take in and accept all our thoughts and feelings as we're aware instead of pushing them away or trying to ignore them mindfulness can enable us to embrace our own selves. In order to deal with difficult thoughts or huge difficulties We always turn to denial, distraction, or reduction. We believe that these thoughts aren't healthy or feelings as we push away our emotions. We acknowledge our ability to manage and all the aspects of us are acceptable as we invite them into our lives.

For instance, we might think of unpleasant emotions such as anger or apathy as a result of the practice of mindfulness.

These aspects of ourselves might not be enjoyable, but they're normal and, once we accept them and embraced, we can learn from and change these aspects. We will not be able to alter our anger or envy when we attempt to remove away these feelings; they are only possible through acceptance. Mindfulness is the choice to concentrate on the present moment. It's not like contemplating our problems or wallowing in our sadness. It's a genuine acceptance of the feelings we're experiencing and who we are.

We don't need to be flawless

We accept the world around us and everybody else as they are, while we are aware. We're not trying to be perfect. We're not trying to be an ideal person. We're not trying to distract attention from our problems. We look at anything without making an opinion on what is good or not. We can let our emotions run wild, however they are, to be, to guide us. We need to remove our glasses and fake faces and stop pretending that everything is going well, even though it's not. We're focusing on what's in our view, and therefore mindfulness is a must. This doesn't mean that we are unaware of the past, or of the future, it's just that we are aware of the benefits and want to live completely only in this moment. Our highest points will be higher and our lows lower, but we're sure they're real and we're not trying to conceal them or transform them into something else.

We relax by tuning in and really listen to the body, our emotions, and thoughts while being conscious; we take note of each aspect of us and accept it. We declare that I am who I am at this moment as well as that I'm a good fit and worthy of my present state.

How to Build Loving Relationships by focusing on Mindfulness

One of the primary indicators of happiness, health and survival is having positive relationships. When we take the time to to know each other and ourselves better, our relationships flourish.

Here are three methods to enhance your existing relationships and help others who need a little help.

Simple ways to strengthen your Relationships

Begin with kindness

A person who is kind attracts another like magnets. People enjoy being around nice people due to feeling cared by them and feel comfortable in their presence. It is said that the Golden Rule still holds true in the present: "Do unto others as you would like them to do to you."

It's also a two-way road. We not only feel better when we exercise compassion, but we also assist others in feeling more positive. As a result we are more likely to engage in meaningful conversations throughout each day. It improves our overall health and wellbeing.

* Be rid of toxic people

Review your relationships to identify who is helping you and who drains you. You'll feel comfortable at ease, secure, and energized in a healthy collaboration.

Once you've determined who's there for you, try to avoid spending time with those who consume you. However, this may not be necessarily the case (i.e. family members or coworkers.) However, in these circumstances, consider how you can improve your friendship by acknowledging that the people may be dealing with the feeling of insecurity that they are experiencing that they face in their lives. Find out what happens when you convert those wishes as a loving-kindness mediation.

• Focus on the similarity instead of variations.

If you're looking to develop a more of a sense of community within your life, think about what we share as fellow human beings, even with people with whom you may not necessarily have a common sense of.

If you are going throughout your daily routine and encounter people who are different from you, simply say "Just like me" and then observe the things you observe. It is possible that you will discover that we all want the same things, namely to be loved and respected and feeling a sense of belonging.

Reactivating your relationship

Routines will eventually become element life in every aspect. They are a part of our daily lives due to a myriad of reasons. They enable us to be more efficient and prevent exhaustion. Routines face the difficulty of being easy and relaxing and spilling out into every aspect that we live, such as our marriages.

We start to think of our companion as a snob and just go through the motions, only to become bored in the end.

* Make use of your relationship the opposite way to benefit

It's wonderful to share a commonality with your partner But opposites do attract. The law of Polarity is the name that has been that is given to this idea. Take the time to think about the first time that you met your beloved. Between you, it was easy and your physical connection demonstrated your instant attraction. Keep in mind the warmth and the chemistry you share as you rekindle your friendship. Maintain your vitality and self-confidence; your wife will continue to be attracted to you at your most natural.

The relationship's chemistry is created by the interactions between your personal energy and that from your spouse. It's not necessary to hide who you are when you interact in a balanced, normal manner, and you are able to be comfortable how you feel. If you're in the situation of needing to rebuild a relationship you'll likely find that one or both of you has lost their authentic self along the process - and the regaining of this vitality is crucial for moving forward.

* Make sure you are physically active to build affection.

When things are difficult and we're trying to revive an affair, many of us struggle to feel physically intimate with our loved ones. This is particularly the case in relationships where sexual intimacy can be a source of contention. It doesn't matter if you're hurting your partner by becoming less close to them or not allowing sex at a particular time and you want to resolve the issue immediately. If one or more of you fail to express affection in a physical way in a meaningful way, it's almost impossible to restore a friendship.

Physical contact regardless of whether it's intimate or not it can provide a normal feeling produced by the body's hormones. This will help you to get into the right state of mind to ignite affection. Be sure to keep in touch with your partner frequently to help you develop feelings of affection and intimacy. Send your loved one an reassuring hug, a gentle kiss or even a simple grasp of your hand to say, "I'm still here and I'm not leaving." If you're trying to repair the bonds of friendship, these simple gestures can make a huge difference to your companion.

Sexuality is a crucial element in relationships and knowing the relationship's sexuality is essential in determining how you can revive the relationship. If you're experiencing an increase in sexual intimacy, but it's declining and you're not sure what to do, it's best to act now before it becomes a major issue.

Be interested in your partner

You were enthralled by your partner as soon as you began to date them. At all times you needed to be aware of the thoughts they had about and experiencing. You asked them about their past experiences as well as their hopes in the near future. Are you truly acting like this? In the absence of a clear answer, it's likely that this is an element of the reason why you're looking for ways you can revive your affection.

Being curious about your friend's behavior involves asking questions and being attentive when they answer. This goes beyond asking about their day, or what they'd like to eat at dinner. Learn how they feel about social events and how their new position influences their future goals and how their career plan has changed. The process of repairing a friendship becomes easier for you all once you have piqued your desire to meet your friend.

* Create and present the most effective effort possible within the team.

Your wife and you are open with each other right from the beginning. Both of you show the best aspects of yourself when you first started meeting. You thought about all the time of methods to impress your partner by making her feel special by creating love messages or planning lavish dinner dates. You were, more than anything the most devoted fan of your partner and they were also yours. How did it end what did this tie in to your desire to know how to renew the relationship?

It's easy to fall into bad habits with your partner and not give the same amount of effort, so don't make the mistake of taking the easy way to your relationship. One of the 10 cardinal guidelines for love is to dedicate yourself to constantly strengthening your relationship. Are you interested in hearing what you can do to revive your romantic relationship?

Be aware that the longevity in your marriage is built on the same principles that led to the first courtship. Remember the things you did to impress your partner. What impact would it have for your friend today if you took an extra few minutes to let them know that they are loved? Be aware that if you are innovative and show a lot of effort to strengthen your bond, it will only grow stronger and develop. If you begin putting effort to a mature relationship right from the beginning the process of fixing a relationship does it by itself.

* Use the conversation as a method of creating an atmosphere of intimacy.

Your words are the same as physical contact and consideration in the course of a relationship. Your words are a major influence and those seeking ways to revive their relationship might not realize how the phrases they've used for their spouse are actually damaging their relationship. The stories we tell ourselves about the person we are and our actions, but they can also strengthen or degrade our partner or relationships. It is not a "right" way to express yourself in all situations. What you must do is be truthful. One example of this is to learn how to ignite romance, and to do this it is necessary to know how to be able to successfully interact with your spouse.

When you're talking with your partner whether it's about your trip to the supermarket or settling a personal disagreement make sure you use genuine words. Make sure you tell them "I love you,"" "thank you,"" and "I love you" along

119

with other phrases. These simple words, said with genuine feelings will make difficult times between you two easier which allows you to create or rebuild faith after having been lost.

Rekindle the love of your life by communicating with sensitivity and care, And, at all cost eliminating blame. If you're having a debate, don't say something that you'll regret later in the midst of it. Remember that this person is someone that you cherish and are able to trust and that your remarks can have a profound impact on the person. It will be apparent that the renewed affection is more profound than the one that you had at the beginning of your relationship. When you join forces to show your admiration and love to one another.

* Resolve conflict through amusement

Don't ignore tension when you're afraid of working on issues while trying to revive the flame of a relationship. When it is handled correctly, conflict can lead to growth, according couples who are committed to improving their relationship. It is important to address the issue before it gets beyond reach and to do it in a way that's relaxing, not stressful.

It's not surprising that you felt like that the world was about to end several times during your high school years when you had to contend with many new experiences and situations. But, now that you're an adult with the advantage of hindsight and experience you may laugh about your "insurmountable" difficulties. It will be easier to figure out ways to reconnect with a friend when you incorporate this "can-do" attitude into your new relationship.

When you're in a heated argument with your partner, just move on to the point at which you're laughing. Keep in mind you can manipulate your mood is a skill that you must master; you do not have to be influenced by your emotions or control them as you discover how to ignite the flame of love. Don't be afraid to confront the issue, instead employ laughter to make it manageable. Consider becoming angry over the situation while doing an outrageous dance or speaking in an animated voice. If you're fighting, you'll learn to tie your partner to positive feelings until you smile and you will.

When handled properly repair of a damaged relationship can be a difficult and exhausting job. You'll be able to navigate through the rough landscape together and create an enjoyable and mutually beneficial friendship if you are able to joke with your companion and connect with humor and laughter.

* Take note of it

Couples may have trouble sharing their feelings face-to-face when trying to ignite passion. It could be due to the fear that the words they speak will impact their partner, anxiety about making the right words or limiting the assumptions they make about their speaking ability. Certain people prefer speaking through writing, particularly during the initial stages of trying to repair the relationship.

Write down your feelings to allow you to express your gratitude and love for your familymembers, offer an understanding apology to deal with painful emotions, and then offer an understanding apology. Once you're finished you can gift the writing to your loved one or keep it to yourself. The goal of the writing is to aid you in recognizing your personal emotions and to find the right words to convey to the person you love.

* Make future ground rules for the future.

What brought you upon the conclusion that you'd like to revive your passion? Do what you can to avoid another similar situation following the time you've restored your confidence and connection. Set guidelines: Do you both desire to put your own and the interests of your relationship above your own? What decisions will be made by each of you individually, and what decisions will be jointly made?

Chapter 7: Borderline Personality Disorder: Take Control Of Impulsions As Well As Mood Swings Using Dbt

The how you feel and think about yourself and other people is affected negatively when you suffer from the disorder known as borderline personality (BPD). It can be a source of stress and makes it difficult to function well in your daily activities. It also causes issues with self-esteem, which can lead to unstable relationships and makes it difficult to control your moods or behavior. The disorder of borderline personality brings the anxiety or fear of being abandoned and may cause anxiety when you are alone. Insanity, insensitive expressions of anger, as well as continuous mood swings could drive people away, even though you wish to develop long-lasting as well-balanced relationships.

Typically, borderline personality disorder is seen in the early years of adulthood and can be better as you the passage of time. It is not necessary to be dissatisfied with yourself if you've got BPD or any other disorder, as DBT is a successful method to deal with this mental health condition. Here are some symptoms and signs of BPD:

* A fear of being abandoned that could force you to take drastic measures to prevent any real or imagined rejection or separation from your loved ones.

* A flurry of stress-induced anxiety and disassociation from reality can last only a few minutes or even for hours.

Changes in your self-image and self identity that cause changes in your values and objectives.

* A continuous pattern of intense and unstable relationships in which you may admire one moment and then suddenly realize that the person isn't worth your time or doesn't deserve your affection.

Participating in dangerous, impulsive behaviors such as reckless driving, excessive eating, drug use alcohol abuse, self-sabotage behaviors.

* Continuous and intense mood swings that be present for hours or even days. There are extreme feelings of anger or anxiety. You may also experience joy.

* The constant feeling of emptiness and helplessness that never goes away.

* Engaging in suicidal ideas or self-injury attempts, typically as a response to fear of being rejected or abandoned.

* Extreme and inappropriate bursts of anger and losing your temper often and fast, or fighting physically.

Take note your self-harming thoughts are causing you to engage in thoughts of self-harm, or having thoughts of suicide, get medical help right away.

DBT is widely used in treatment of borderline personality disorder. It is the only type of psychotherapy confirmed to be effective when treating BPD in controlled clinical trials. It is considered to be the standard of treatment for BPD. DBT has been shown as effective at minimizing drug abuse, reducing anxiety about suicide as well as destructive behavior and decreasing the requirement for psychiatric hospitalization. The root of the issue is emotional dysregulation. problem that causes borderline personality disorder. It's often by genetic risk factors as well as genetic risk factors, as well as the unstable environment that affects emotional health in the early years of life or unhealthy methods to manage chronic stress.

The ability to manage your impulses and regulate mood swings is crucial when managing an affliction called bipolar disorder. Here are some tips that can be helpful.

Information on BPD

Begin collecting all the information you can about BPD as you can. When you know what the condition can be and the ways it may be affecting you, it will become simpler to manage it. If you do not know the issues you face it is impossible to manage this disorder. It is also important to start discussing BPD with those you love. A solid support system is a huge boost to the likelihood of being able to manage as well as manage BPD. Be aware that BPD like all other things can be described as the spectrum. When you do this, don't presume that you are the only one. It is always different between people. The typical symptoms that accompany it do not last and it is easily controlled. Don't let the diagnosis be a burden to you. Even in the worst of times you must recognize that it's the BPD which is driving your actions. Once you recognize this, it's much easier to manage BPD.

Take your time and think about your choices

Take a moment to think about all the decisions you've made in the past and especially those associated with your relationships you have in your life. In some instances, you might have been harsh or made rash choices which could result in the loss of several excellent relationships. When you begin to analyze the history of your relationships and identifying any negative patterns of thinking which led you to act unintentionally. Once you recognize these patterns, you'll be more prepared to face like situations again in the near future. It is also never enough to apologize. If you believe you are in the wrong, you must immediately issue an apology. It will reduce the guilt you feel and you'll feel better about yourself.

Don't Cover It Up

There is no need to hide your BPD or attempt to disguise it. Do not let anyone else convince you that you are not. You don't need to conform to the social mold and adhere to any societal rules that don't fit your needs. Individuals are free to express their own opinions, and everyone will see things differently. Do not try to convince yourself that all is well even when you're not feeling well. Accept the fact that you have BPD and learn from it. Once you are able to accept the diagnosis, it can lead to your personal development. Anything that didn't appear to be logical will become clear. You will be able to understand your actions and understand why you live your life what it is. Be open about the subject of BPD with those you love and make them aware of what you're going through. Once they are aware of what you're going through you will be better prepared to manage your emotional reactions. Be aware that your BPD doesn't define you, and it's not your responsibility. Do not blame yourself and refrain from any form of negative thinking.

Use a Journal

An easy way to detach from your emotions and ease your burden of emotional stress is to take note of your emotions. Keep your personal "emotion diary" or diary in which you can share your thoughts out. Sometimes, it is difficult to communicate your feelings to you, or even to your family members. In these instances, get your journal and begin recording what you are feeling. Don't make yourself feel guilty for the words you write. Do not try to analyse them. Instead, see it as a way to express your feelings. When you read what you've written, you will be able to recognize your emotions. Once you have a clear understanding of your feelings and can respond accordingly. It also provides the time to think about your self and reflect. In addition recording your thoughts and feelings is an excellent method to stimulate your mind. Instead of focusing on certain issues, write them down and find the right solutions.

Learn to Know Your Mental State

The ability to focus is crucial to DBT. Knowing how you feel can help you manage your emotions and control them. The three states of mind that are part of DBT include: reasonable mind, emotional mind and the wise mind. When you are in a rational mind, you are likely to take things in a rational manner and plan your actions and pay attention to all information you can get, and respond in a manner that is appropriate. This could be that is as easy as measuring ingredients prior to cooking. A rational mind allows you to remain in the right direction and remain rational.

The mind of the emotional however is driven by emotions. The logic of thinking is thrown out of the window and the truth can be easily altered. This mental state typically leads to impulsive behavior and negative thoughts patterns. For example, going on an unexpected trip or fighting with someone because you aren't both in agreement on a certain subject. When you understand your emotional mind it can be easy to find ways that you could be hurting yourself in a way that isn't intentional. If your rational mind and your emotional mind join together, they are referred to by the term "wise mind. It's about the feeling of intuition or a feeling that something is isn't quite correct. Maybe you feel an innate sense that something isn't quite right , or you experience something that can't be described with your mind's logical thinking.

When you experience a desire to react, think about the mindset you're in and you can enhance your reactions to events.

Examine the information

There are two easy actions you can take when trying to manage BPD These are called "checking factual information." If you are experiencing extreme stress or anxiety be sure to verify the facts before you react or react to an event. It is the first thing to recognize the emotion you feel. Next, you must determine whether the emotion you are feeling is legitimate by looking up all the information or facts available regarding the emotion you're experiencing. If you believe that your reactions aren't appropriate or you're reacting in a way that is impulsive, consider taking a step back to relax before reacting. This is a crucial capability that will help you in many areas that you face in life.

Positive Self-Talk

If you're looking to be able to control your reactions to various circumstances and react with a healthy attitude now is the time to change your negative reactions or habits by using positive self-talk. It's going to take time and effort to master it. If you focus in positive thoughts about yourself, you will be able to ease anxiety, boost your focus, and remain more focused. Be sure to remind yourself that you're worthy of everything that is that are good and beautiful in this world. Instead of dwelling over the negative thoughts that you think of about your life or the people around you, think about positive things. Every moment in your life is fleeting and nothing is permanent. The only constant is change in the world. So, even the most difficult of experiences will be over. What is the point in wasting your precious energy and time thinking about all the unpleasant events even if they're just temporary? Remember that what that you're in doesn't define your present or your future. The future is not yours to control as it is unpredictably unpredictable. Doing anything about it will only make you feel more stressed. Instead of thinking about the past focus on the things you can do to change the situation the next time you encounter it. It allows you to have more control over your behavior and actions, rather than feeling like you're being in a position of being a victim.

Reframe all negative thoughts with positive self-talk. For example, if a presentation did not go as planned you may think to your self, "I am a failure and can't succeed in anything." Instead of thinking about negative events then you could think "The presentation didn't take the direction I had hoped for it to. I can speak to my colleagues and find the areas in which I have to make improvements." When you are aware of the negative self-talk you are putting into your head and replacing it with positive thoughts You can control your mood.

Check-In with Youself

The health of your body is your own responsibility. There is no one else who can help you with it and, unless you take good care of yourself and your health, you will not be able to manage BPD. Distress and anger are typically the typical reactions to any situation or circumstance in which you suffer from BPD. For example, if a acquaintance did something that upset you, your first reaction could be to yell at the person or even threaten to harm the person. Instead of this do a quick take a moment to check in with yourself. When you've done this, you will be able to effectively convey your feelings to the person you are talking to in a non-threatening way. Through the simple practice of mindfulness it is possible to avoid relationships from going south. In addition, you'll be more adept at managing your thoughts and emotions.

If for example, your companion was late to your scheduled date, your first reaction could be to become angry. Your typical reaction is to shout at him and question why he's rude or inconsiderate towards you. Before doing that you should take a moment to examine yourself. Determine your primary and secondary emotions. In this case, you're likely angry or frustrated because you're afraid that your spouse doesn't care or you are worried about the issues with abandonment you may have.

After you've identified the feelings, you can inquire with the reason why he is late. It is certainly the best way to deal the situation.

Chapter 8: Who Can Benefit From Dbt?

DBT is particularly effective for those who feel emotional reactions that are intense. They can be overwhelmed by the demands of life and relationship stressors until they feel like their emotional reactions are out of hand. Therefore, they tend to react in a impulsive way to try to temporarily ease some of the stress. But, their actions in the long run result in more problems.

DBT was originally developed to aid people who were identified with Borderline Personality Disorder (BPD.) It has proven to be an extremely efficient therapy for this group of people. In more recent times, DBT has also been extensively used for people who have intense mood swings and who are not able to implement strategies for coping with these sudden and intense emotional impulses. A lot of them struggle with serious depression PTSD as well as eating disorders as well as severe compulsory disorders. Bipolar Disorder ADHD and anger control and addiction issues. A large portion of those who seek DBT may also be self-harming since this method has been proven highly effective in helping those suffering from this kind of emotional distress.

To know more about the individual who excels in DBT Let's examine the particular characteristics that a lot of them have. The people who excel in DBT typically are prone to high levels of vulnerability to emotional issues. This means that they tend to experience emotions in a very receptive and intense manner. Sometimes, they're just wired to experience emotions more strongly than people of average age. In reality, DBT theory asserts that the Automatic Nervous System of an vulnerable person who is emotionally vulnerable is more likely to react to small level of stress. The nervous system of these people also is slower to recover to its normal state after the stressor is gone in comparison to other people. In addition, certain people suffer from mood disorders like Major Depression or Generalized Anxiety which are not effectively controlled by medications that alter the intensity of their emotions. Therefore, people who are emotionally vulnerable tend to experience quick emotional, intense reactions which are difficult to control. They are in a trance through their entire lives.

However, doctors have discovered that those who are the most emotionally vulnerable seeking DBT treatment are not wired to experience more intense emotions or suffer from mood disorders. They are often exposed to situations which were not a valid one for long period of time, generally starting in the early years of childhood, but could happen at any time. These environments didn't offer them the help with respect, attention or understanding they required to deal with their feelings. The effects of invalidating environments be anything from extreme physical or emotional abuse to the incompatible parents and children's personalities. Think about the shy child who was either adopted or born into a household that is full of extroverts, and who is constantly being teased about the introverted side of him. Perhaps it's the child who suffers from ADHD who has a mom as well as a stepfather that are rigid and always yelling at her. Both are instances of situations which are blaming. If someone who is predisposed to experiencing more intense emotions is placed in a situation which does not allow or affirm his feelings, he may be more vulnerable emotionally. Then, he may begin to show more emotional reactivity as he accidentally discovers that the only moment when he's considered to be a serious threat is when he displays this extreme emotion.

Let's use the child who is introverted as an illustration. Imagine that he was continually being told by his father that he needed be able to "man into the world" and be more assertive in his attitude to life. He was ridiculed and began to think it was something amiss in his character. One day, as his father was talking to him, the child began crying uncontrollably. The father instantly slowed down and his mother ran to help him to shower him with lots of love. It happened again. And again. A fascinating thing started to unfold. The child's mind started to recognize patterns that resembled this: My father yells at me, I yell uncontrollably until the screaming stops, I am surrounded by attention. The boy begins to do this every day because it's effective, and each successful display inadvertently strengthens the behaviour. His emotional outbursts have been recognized and it eventually becomes a habitual coping technique.

The behavior described above, subconsciously heightened the child's vulnerability to emotional trauma and guessed what was a lot more difficult. This is a common kind of pattern that is seen in those suffering from the condition known as Borderline Personality Disorder, Bipolar Disorder, eating disorders, and various other disorders related to the disorders that DBT treats. The following section will provide an overview of many of the disorders that can be successfully treated using DBT therapies.

Borderline Personality Disorder

People who have BPD suffer from a variety of issues. Disorder (BPD) are prone to experiencing emotions more intensely and over longer time periods than the rest of us. They are more susceptible to frequent and frequent outbursts in such a way that Mental Health professionals have described this group as having a constant stress. They're nearly always in crisis as they are not generally taught the coping strategies they require to control their emotional turmoil.

The people suffering from BPD are more vulnerable to emotional trauma and they take longer to recover to their the baseline after an incident. Furthermore one of the underlying characteristics that Therapists have identified about people suffering from BPD is that they tend to adopt the same beliefs system as the shaming environment they are a part of. This causes "self-invalidation" in which they deny their own feelings and abilities to resolve issues. They also develop unrealistic expectations for themselves , and feel a sense of shame and frustration when they fail to achieve their goals or when problems develop.

A further characteristic that distinguishes people who suffer from BPD is the tendency they have to create rigid and unattainable expectations of their own and other. If things don't go according to the way they'd like, or as they'd like They often turn towards "blaming." The habit of blaming others is an unthinking error that many people suffering from BPD suffer from. They blame everything and everyone for their issues and struggle to acknowledge the behavioral changes they are required to notice the different results in their lives.

People with BPD suffer from a lack of self-esteem and tend to struggle with relationships. They are more likely to look for people who can take charge and resolve their issues for them, so they can retreat and not be forced to deal with it. They also cover themselves in a mask of competence so that people believe they can solve their own issues and managing their intense emotions. Although they've been able to master certain aspects of their lives however, they haven't had success in extending their abilities in other areas of their lives.

Due to the life style that the majority of people with BDP have created, along with their inability to return to normal following an emotional experience They are prone to experiencing traumatizing experiences that are significant over and over again. They also have a tendency to avoid having negative emotions altogether since they don't know how to control even positive negative emotions. In the end, they don't know the best way to respond when an emotion circumstance is encountered that they are unable to handle, which can lead them into a heightened and long-lasting emotional state.

People who suffer from Borderline Personality Disorder can take part in cutting, or self-harm, as well as suicidal actions to ease the extreme emotional pain. The vulnerability of the emotional is frequently seen in those who are suicidal or who engage in chronic self-injury. The person is emotional and, when exposed to trauma that is extremely severe, like emotional or physical abuse, she may consider suicide. In the end, as a way to ease the constant pain she decides to commit suicide and is admitted to the hospital. There she receives a lot of attention , and for the first time, she starts to feel that she is receiving recognition and being taken seriously.

Think about the child who commits a type self-injury like burning or cutting himself because it gives him temporary relief. When someone else learns the incident the world suddenly starts to take his actions seriously. Similar to what happened to this girl described in the earlier instance, this is the first time, he's finally feeling accepted.

What are your thoughts on what is happening in these two scenarios? In time, remain engaged in the actions because it's the only way they feel valued and accepted. It becomes a deeply ingrained ability.

Disorders of Eating

A disorder of eating is a disease which is marked by eating patterns that are irregular. However, the disease extends beyond a simple change in food intake , as the individual suffering from the disorder typically is in a state of extreme distress about their body's weight and/or appearance. In order to control your appearance, and also feel more confident at their best, people suffering from eating disorders can start eating less, and may become obsessed with exercising. This behavioral and emotional disorder is common in males and females, and is extremely detrimental on the emotional and physical health of the person.

Although eating disorders can develop at any stage of development however, they typically manifest at the adolescent or early adulthood , and frequently occurs in conjunction with other behavioral and psychological conditions like addiction disorders, anxiety as well as mood disorder. The three most frequent kinds of eating Disorders comprise Anorexia Nervosa as well as Bulimia Nervosa as well as Binge Eating Disorder. We will explain each disorder in greater depth below.

Anorexia Nervosa:

Anorexics who suffer from Nervosa often has an intense anxiety about their weight. Because of their distorted and unrealistic impressions of their body they are afraid of weight gain and tend to avoid maintaining the weight of a healthy body. A lot of people suffering from Anorexia Nervosa reduce the amount of food they consume to the extent they is not enough to support their health. Even when they appear to be underweight and their appearance is beginning to cause concern among others, they think of themselves as overweight. Anorexia can cause serious health issues, such as organ failure, brain damage and bone loss heart issues, infertility. The risk of dying is greatest for people suffering from this disorder.

Bulimia Nervosa:

People who suffer from Bulimia typically fear being overweight and feel unhappy with their bodies. This condition is characterised with the pattern of eating excessively followed by an overcompensation to the excessive eating. For instance, one might eat large quantities of food in one sitting. They may after eating, they will follow it up by vomiting forcefully, excessive exercise, excessive diuretics and laxatives and any other combination of compensatory behavior. The whole process takes place in secret since they typically have a lot of guilt, shame and feelings of a lack of control over their behavior. The condition can cause health issues such as digestive issues, dehydration, as well as heart problems that are caused by an imbalance in electrolytes caused by the purging of food.

Binge Eating Disorder:

The people who experience Binge Eating tend to lose control of their food intake, but don't take part in the process of purging as is the case with Bulimia. Therefore, many who suffer from Binge Eating might also suffer from the condition of obesity that can lead to health problems like heart disease. Similar to those who suffer from different eating disorders those who suffer from this disorder typically experience feelings of deep guilt, shame as well as embarrassment. They also feel a sense of a lack of control.

The process of development of eating disorders can be multi-faceted because the causes are very complicated. Certain factors can contribute to the emergence of eating disorders.

The causes of an eating disorder for an individual is an array of psychological, biological and, of course, environmental factors. The factors that can cause an eating disorder include:

* Genetic factors like abnormal hormone functions, as well as an inherited predisposition.

* Nutritional deficiencies

* Psychological aspects such as a bad body image or a negative self-esteem

* Environmental influences like:

• Dysfunctional unit of the family

* Careers and professions that encourage excessively thinness such as modeling

* Sports that require a certain degree of the idea of being thin for performance, such as wrestling, gymnastics long distance running and more.

* Child sexual abuse

* Peer pressure, family pressure and media pressure to look thin

* Life transitions and changes

Here are a few signs and symptoms one might exhibit when they are struggling in an eating disorder.

* Frequent and extreme eating, even when extremely underweight

• Obsession over caloric consumption as well as the amount of fat in food items.

* Demonstrating ritualistic eating practices. This could include actions like cutting food into small pieces, eating with a partner and storing food items to be consumed later.

* A fixation of food. Individuals with eating disorders can cook delicious, intricate meals for their friends but are unable to eat.

People with eating disorders might also be suffering from depression or lethargy.

While DBT has been proven to be highly effective in treating patients suffering from eating Disorders However, patients may require extra support during the initial stages of treatment , too. The additional support could include monitoring by a doctor to address all health problems that might be developing, as well as working with a nutritionist until the weight has stabilized. The Nutritionist often develops an individual diet plan that helps those who are struggling to maintain an ideal weight.

Bipolar Disorder

Bipolar Disorder is sometimes called Manic Depressive Disorder due to the patient's tendency to oscillate between manic and depressive state. This condition is characterised by extreme and unpredictably extreme changes in energy levels, mood as well as activity levels and the capacity to complete daily activities. The symptoms differ from normal mood changes since they are severe and often quite extreme in the sense that people generally damage relationships, impede the performance of their school and work or even consider suicide at time or two.

Like many mental illnesses there is no one cause that is the sole reason for Bipolar

Disorder. It's often a condition that is caused by a mix of environmental and biological causes. Numerous factors interact to trigger the illness or increase the likelihood of it appearing.

Genetics is believed to influence the rise of Bipolar Disorder, as studies have identified a few genes more likely to contribute to the formation that cause the condition. Another study has revealed that children who come from certain families or who have siblings with Bipolar Disorder are at a higher risk to be affected by the disorder in their own.

However, studies have revealed the influence of environmental variables on an important part in the development of the disorder also. In studies of identical twins in which siblings share identical genetic characteristics in which one twin develops the disorder, the other is not always affected by the disorder , as expected given their identical genetic composition. This suggests that something other than genetics is responsible that could be due at environmental triggers.

Patients with Bipolar Disorder suffer from extreme emotional states, which are known as "mood episode." The episodes could last for days or even months before it is over. Each episode shows a significant alteration in the normal behavior of the patient. A wildly joyful, exuberant state filled with activity is often described as a "manic" incident. The despairing, sad or hopeless and occasionally angry and explosive state is known as the "depressive incident." An "mixed situation" is when the characteristics of both manic episodes and an episode of depression occur simultaneously.

Here are a few symptoms that can be attributed to Bipolar Disorder:

Manic episodes can manifest as symptoms like:

* A prolonged duration of experiencing "high" that is reflected by an exuberantly happy or a jovial mood

* Talking extremely fast and moving between ideas. This is indicative of racing thoughts.

It is easy to get distracted.

• Excessive activity and taking on numerous new projects

* Unrest

* Sleeping is limited

Unrealistic ideas about the possibilities one has

* Impulsivity and obsession with exciting and risky pursuits

The symptoms of a depression episode are:

* prolonged periods of extreme irritation

• Long days of depressing sadness or despair

• Loss of interest in the activities once loved

* Feeling tired and sluggish

* Troubles concentrating, remembering and making decisions

* Changes in eating habits, sleeping, or other routines

* Suicidal ideas, behaviors and/or suicidal ideas could be present

Bipolar Disorder may be present in a person, at times when their moods aren't so than extreme. In particular, sufferers of Bipolar Disorder have hypomania which is a milder kind of the disorder known as mania. In a hypomanic episode the patient may feel extremely well and may even be efficient. Although they may be performing perfectly, their family and friends are noticing a dramatic shift in mood. The changes in mood are so striking that family members and friends might be wondering whether symptoms from Bipolar Disorder are present. Without treatment it is possible for hypomania to develop into full-blown mania, or signs associated with Bipolar Disorder may occur.

As we have mentioned before, Bipolar Disorder may be present in an unipolar state. This occurs when a person is experiencing depression and mania simultaneously. When in a mixed state it is possible to feel extremely stressed, suffer from sleep disruption or significant changes in appetite and might even be prone to suicidal thoughts. People who are in a mixed state might feel extremely sad or depressed while also feeling very energetic.

If one is experiencing a prolonged episode of depression or mania individuals may suffer from psychotic symptoms, such as hallucinations, delusions or hallucinations and. Psychotic symptoms usually be a reflection of and strengthen the person's extremely mood. For instance, if a person experiencing psychotic symptoms in an episode of manic, they might believe that he's the president of a nation that is wealthy, money, or has some sort of special power. A person experiencing psychotic symptoms during a depression period could be characterized by believing that one is homeless, broken and penniless, or even a criminal in hiding. In reality, many people suffering from Bipolar Disorder are misdiagnosed with Schizophrenia or another reality-testing disorders due to the hallucinations that they experience due to their mood.

Individuals suffering from Bipolar Disorder may also suffer from the co-occurring disorder dependency or poly-substance abuse. Anxiety disorders, like post-traumatic stress Disorder (PTSD) or fears, are often co-occurring. Bipolar Disorder also sometimes co-occurs with Attention Deficit Hyperactivity disorder (ADHD.) Individuals with Bipolar Disorder also tend to be at greater chance of suffering from thyroid diseases headaches caused by migraine, heart diseases, obesity, diabetes and other physical diseases.

Chapter 9: Dbt Tactics And Methods

DBT employs a variety of strategies and techniques which include:

The Heart of Mindfulness

Learning to develop mindfulness skills is a key benefit of DBT.4 Mindfulness allows you to focus on the present moment as well as "live in the present moment," and allows you to pay attention to what's happening inside you (your feelings, thoughts feelings, impulses, and sensations) as well as what's happening in the world around you (what you hear, see, smell, and feel) without judgment.

If you're struggling with anxiety, mindfulness techniques can help you relax and concentrate on using secure methods of coping. The practice will assist in calming your mind and avoid destructive thoughts as well as impulsive behaviors.

Distress Tolerance

The skills of distress tolerance aid you to accept your situation and the present.

You'll be taught four strategies to deal with the stress of a crisis:

* can be a source of distraction

* Adding to the existing situation

* Self-relaxation

Think about the benefits as well as the disadvantages to not being able to tolerate the pain.

Strategies to manage stress can assist you in preparing for difficult emotions and help you manage these feelings in a positive approach in the long term.

Effective Interpersonal Relationships

Effective interpersonal communication allows you to assert yourself more in the context of a relationship (for instance, by speaking up about your needs and telling "no") and while maintaining a positive and stable relationship. You'll increase your listening and communication skills and also your capacity to deal with people who are difficult and respect your own self and those around you.

Emotion Regulation

Controlling your emotions allows you to handle intense emotions with greater ease. The skills you develop can assist you in recognizing the signs, naming and changing your emotions.

It helps reduce your anxiety about emotions and helps you enjoy greater positive interactions with your emotions because you identify and manage powerful negative emotions (for instance anger, for example).

What issues can dialectical Behavioral Therapy help with?

The Dr. Marsha Linehan and colleagues created DBT in the late 1980s following the discovery the fact that cognitive behavioral therapy (CBT) alone didn't perform as effectively as it was intended for people suffering from BPD. The Dr. Linehan and her contemporaries modified strategies and developed the treatment that would meet the needs of these patients.

DBT can be helpful in the following circumstances:

* (ADHAD) Attention-deficit/hyperactivity disorder (ADHD)

* Bipolar disorder

* (BPD)Borderline personality disorder

"Eating Disorders" (Like anorexia nervosaor eating disorder with binge and bulimia nervosa)

* (GAD) Generalized anxiety disorder

* Major depressive disorder (including treatment-resistant major depression and severe depression)

* Non-suicidal self-injury

* (OCD) Obsessive-compulsive disorder

* (PTSD) Post-traumatic stress disorder

* Use of substances in disorder

* Suicidal behavior

The benefits of Dialectical Behavioral Therapy

163

In DBT the patient and their psychiatrist work together to work through the perception of conflict between self-acceptance as well as improvement to aid recovering patients achieve significant improvements. Giving validation is an integral part of this method that makes people more likely to be involved and less anxious about the thought of a transition.

In reality, the psychiatrist affirms that the individual's choices "make sense" considering their personal experience but doesn't believe that they are the only way to resolve the problem.

Although the design and goals of each treatment setting differ, DBT features can be observed in group skill instruction as well as individual psychotherapy and telephone coaching.1

Change and acceptance Learning ways to accept and tolerate the experiences of your life, your feelings as well as yourself. You'll also acquire abilities which will aid you in improving your relationships and behavior with other people.

Behavior: You'll learn how to recognize challenges and bad behaviors, and then replace them with more healthy and successful ones.

Cognitive: You'll focus to alter harmful or ineffective beliefs and habits, attitudes and behaviors.

Collaboration: You'll learn to collaborate effectively and successfully in groups (therapist or group therapist or psychiatrist).

Skills: You'll acquire new abilities through learning new techniques.

Support: You'll feel energized to look at and nurture your qualities and strengths.

Effectiveness

Individuals may be taught better ways to manage and express emotions with this therapy method because it helps them build their coping abilities. DBT is effective regardless of age, background and gender or sexual orientation or race/ethnicity according to research.

165

DBT is beneficial in treating borderline personality disorder as well as in reducing the chance of suicide in those suffering from BPD according to research. According to one study greater than 75% those who suffer from BPD do not have the diagnostic criteria for the disorder after one year of treatment.

A second study revealed that treatments that included skills training as a feature of therapy proved more effective than DBT without skill training in the prevention of suicide.

For mental health issues that are not listed Although the majority of DBT literature has been devoted to its application for people with borderline personality disorder, who exhibit suicidal and self-injury tendencies, the method is also beneficial to those with mental health concerns.

This kind of therapy, as an example can be found to be successful for treating PTSD stress, PTSD, and anxiety, as per research studies.

Think about the below

DBT requires a significant time investment. It is expected that people do "homework" as well as regular therapy sessions that focus on their skills, which is not only in the group, individual, and phone counseling sessions. If you have difficulty staying on top of these activities on a regular basis it could be a concern.

For some people, attempting certain skills could be challenging. Some people are exposed to painful events and physical discomfort at different levels of recovery. This can be stressful.

How to Begin

It is the only method to know whether DBT is a good fit the best treatment for your needs is to discuss with a trained expert in DBT. To determine whether DBT is a suitable fit for you, they'll take a look at your symptoms, your treatment history and treatment objectives.

If you or someone close to you believes that DBT might be helpful, consult to a doctor or mental health professional who has been trained in the method. But finding DBT therapists can be difficult.

The Clinical Resource Directory, hosted by the Behavioral Tech is an excellent starting point for your search (an organization that was founded by Dr. Linehan to train mental health professionals in DBT). The directory lets you search by state for therapists and other services that have been through DBT instruction from the Behavioral Tech LLC in conjunction with the University of Washington's Behavioral Therapy Clinics.

You can also ask for an appointment with a friend who is an expert in DBT through your physician or new psychiatrist or another well-respected mental health professional. DBT Therapists that offer online counseling services are also available.

Chapter 10: Exposure Therapy

Anxious Fears

Exposure therapy is an CBT technique that can be used to aid those suffering from anxiety issues and phobias. The study of this method has been conducted by a qualified practitioner, it's both reliable and safe.

The use of exposure therapy is primarily to treat:

*Post-Traumatic Stress Disorder (PTSD)

* Panic attacks

* Obsessive-compulsive disorder (OCD)

* Social Anxiety Disorder (SAD)

*Generalized Anxiety Disorder (GAD)

The background of exposure therapy goes back to before CBT. It began as a form of treatment that was prescribed by psychologists who dealt with behavioral issues. The basis for this was built in classical conditioning. The most well-known study of classical conditioning was

Pavlov's experiments with dogs. Pavlov trained dogs to salivate upon any sound in order to prepare them for with the addition of foods.

Behavioral psychologists, like B.F. Skinner, took this concept to the next level. The concept of operant conditioning was a different way of altering certain behavior. Skinner believed that behavior was determined by its consequences which were good or not. The consequences determine whether the behavior is continued or not. Positive consequences reinforce the behavior. While negative consequences could, for the majority of people, lead to the end of this behaviour.

The person who came up with the idea is Mary Cover Jones, often called the founder of the field of behavior therapy, who pioneered the notion of desensitization. It's a method that involves repeatedly exposing a patient to the trigger that may be the source of anxiety. This is commonly referred to as exposure therapy.

Fear is an intense emotion. If we are scared of something, it's normal that we want to stay away from it. In certain circumstances, it's acceptable, like when you shouldn't meet a bear in a planned way. In a more real-world setting there are people who might be afraid to drive at a high speed, so stay clear of this scenario. Another common and sensible fear. When your fears concentrate on more ordinary circumstances that it's thought to be a risky kind of anxiety. Maybe you are in an enclosed area, or in crowds. Avoiding situations that are commonplace could have a negative impact on the quality of your life. Refraining from situations that cause you to feel sick, might at first seem like the right option. It's a good idea to alleviate your anxiety. What it is actually doing is actually causing the anxiety. If you don't confront the fear that is causing you anxiety it is impossible to overcome it.

The goal of exposure therapy is stopping the habit of avoidance to ensure that it is not as ad hoc. This kind of therapy comes with different techniques. They are customized by the therapist to meet the needs of the client.

Common Exposure Methods

In-Vivo Exposure

A treatment plan that directs the patient to the stimulus. The procedure is performed by a certified therapy therapist. It is about confronting the anxiety. A good example is someone who suffers from an insufferable fears of flying. One of the aspects of treatment might involve them going to an airport before taking a flight. The patient will not be on their own as they will be accompanied by a certified professional. Throughout the course, the patient is advised to use calm techniques, like controlled breathing.

Interoceptive Exposure

A technique in which the therapist creates physical sensations. The aim is to encourage the patient to contemplate and write about their fears. These physical sensations could be characterized by a shortening of breath tension in the muscles, or the rapid heartbeat. This is the intention of proving that these physical sensations, though uncomfortable, aren't risky.

Imagineal Exposure

Sometimes, it is used in a similar manner In a way, it is often used in conjunction with In Vivo Exposure. It differs from In Vivo Exposure in that it employs Imaginal Exposure. The patient isn't exposed directly to the event that triggers anxiety. They are instead urged to imagine the fear that caused them anxiety. As with Interoceptive Exposure, the intent is to trigger emotions of anxiety.

Virtual Reality Exposure

This is a brand new method. It involves putting the patient into an immersive virtual environment typically using headsets. It is an ideal way to expose an individual to specific situations they consider to be unsafe within the actual world. Particularly beneficial for those suffering PTSD and has proved successfully used in working with combat veterans.

A key aspect of exposure therapy is to determine the amount of exposure to the anxious stimuli. Overexposure too early could be harmful to the client. There are three ways of determining the amount of exposure in CBT.

Systematic Desensitization

Exposure to stimuli that can cause anxiety when engaging in activities to reduce stress. This could include breathing exercises like controlled breathing or other relaxation methods.

Gradually Exposed Exposure

With the assistance of the counselor, the client is asked to create an orderly list of anxious situations. The treatment involves exposure to most threatening fears first. Then, the build-up to the more challenging scenarios gradually.

Flooding

The method is more violent and somewhat controversial approach to exposure therapy. This is due to the fact that this technique can cause anxiety by overwhelming the patient with stimuli. Although it can only be utilized on a select number of patients however, it's the most efficient and cost-effective method. It has been shown to treat anxiety, phobias, and other problems.

Does the therapy of exposure works?

There have been an abundance of research that shows this type of therapy works in helping individuals suffering from anxiety problems. The extent to which it works for every individual is contingent on the approach of the therapist. A study conducted of Rothbaum & Schwartz (2002) (5a) shows that it's effective in the treatment of PTSD. In the majority of cases, a gradual approach is essential to successful treatment. If the patient isn't rushed into it and is taken each step by itself and the patient is able to beat the fear that they experience.

Here are a few examples of how various techniques of exposure therapy could assist in the treatment of the symptoms of PTSD:

PTSD sufferers may have suffered from an event that was traumatizing or experienced one. The typical symptoms of PTSD may include recurring alarming thoughts and terrifying nightmares. While they replay the experience over and over again in their mind and experience the trauma, they become more vigilant, (always on the lookout for danger). All of these signs could lead to depression.

Like many anxiety-related issues sufferers with PTSD are able to use the same method to find relief, which is usually avoidance. This isn't a good thing, as avoidance increases the anxiety and it could lead to additional issues. The additional problems can be an emotional disconnect from people around you or even family members. Together with a lack of enthusiasm for life, and the possibility of depression. Therapy for exposure to PTSD may take various forms. Utilizing the various methods that we've mentioned previously look at how they are incorporated into an PTSD patient's treatment:

In-Vivo Exposure

Patient is exposed to incident that triggers the anxiety. This could include visiting the location of the traumatizing incident. For instance, someone who was victim of an incident that was violent could go to the location where it occurred. A professional therapist will help them to confront the feelings that are triggered. This must be a controlled circumstance as the patient could be overwhelmed and need to leave the area immediately.

Imagineal Exposure

If the patient isn't yet ready to confront the reality of the incident it is the best option. In this case, the patient employs imaginative techniques to recreate the traumatizing experience. It is essential to replay the events in their minds. Together with the help of a trained therapist who can assist them in challenging the thoughts and emotions that the memory brings to.

Interoceptive Exposure

A common sign of PTSD may manifest as panic attack. These attacks usually occur caused by a physical sensation, like the sensation of a heart racing or breath shortness. Through this method, the therapist attempts to trigger those feelings. This is achieved by encouraging the patient hyperventilate. This can be done together with Imagined Exposure. The patient does not only imagine the incident, but also experiencing hyperventilation induced. A study conducted by Wald & Taylor (2008) (5b) confirms it is true that Interoceptive Exposure is effective in alleviating the anxiety of PTSD sufferers.

Virtual Reality Exposure

This approach is becoming more sought-after. It is particularly effective in treating veterans of the armed forces and active soldiers. The condition known as PTSD that is caused by the trauma of war. It's about reliving anxious situations, but without putting the person in physical danger. It can be as simple as immersing the user in an immersive virtual world created by powerful computers. The user is not just immersed in an immersive visual experience, but other senses as well. It may include audio and, sometimes, the sense of tactile sensations. The audio and visual signals are transmitted through headsets. While the sensory experience is perceived by sensors located around the body of the patient. Similar to all exposure therapy methods, the aim is to expose the patient repeatedly to the stimuli that trigger anxiety. In the end, the autonomic response which is the cause in panic attacks, is reduced. This is called "habituation." Virtual Reality Exposure has shown to be effective in aiding PTSD sufferers. It can help reduce the degree symptoms of PTSD symptoms.

Exposure therapy can be a helpful instrument those suffering from PTSD. It also helps with other anxiety disorders like phobias and Obsessive Compulsive Disorders. The different techniques provide ways to challenge the dysfunctional thinking process. In the end it assists patients be able to accept the trauma that triggered the condition in the initial place. The roots of this kind of therapy stem from earlier forms of behavioral psychology. However, like Virtual Reality Exposure, it was developed to assist patients tackle modern-day problems. This is all made possible by the latest modern technology.

Conclusion

Addicts need to learn methods to deal with stress situations without getting lost in their thoughts, without self-judging. It is equally important to be aware of the health issues that addiction can cause. Certain medical conditions can cause an individual to end their life. Most addiction-related effects are harmful, like addiction to drugs and alcohol. They can be psychological or physical impacts. Human bodies, when exposed to substances quickly adjusts in the body's physiological state.

This is why it's more effective to recognize signs of addiction in the initial stages, so that they can be taken care of as soon as is possible. The rate of addiction to porn is increasing among teenagers and young people which is why it is important to be aware of it and the ways to assist addicts at the beginning of addiction. The use of dialectical behavior therapy could be an important solution to addiction porn because the problem of addiction to porn is multi-faceted.

In dealing with addiction Dialectical behavior therapy is a method of dealing with addiction that offers a more sensible approach to understanding and defeating the different kinds of addiction. The power that it offers Dialectical treatment is that it's that it is based in the concept of cognitive behavior which is seen as a method to use cognitive behavioral therapy. It encourages the involvement of addicts.

When it comes to this type of therapy, it's essential that the therapy be executed to the smallest aspect by a highly competent person in order to increase the chances of effectiveness. The effectiveness of the therapy session is determined through the client and counselor forming a cooperative relationship, and it is important to be noted that therapy is not a requirement for all people, even though it's general and is applicable to anyone struggling with different kinds of addiction.

www.ingramcontent.com/pod-product-compliance
Lightning Source LLC
Chambersburg PA
CBHW060333030426
42336CB00011B/1318